MAKE YOURSELF OVER

This is a book aimed at everyone's twin goals:
How to look *and* feel better. No matter what
your age or sex, it's never too late—or too early—
to begin.

Here are the scientifically proven
SECRETS OF HEALTH & BEAUTY
that tell you all you need to know to look and
to feel vitally alive—physically and mentally.
Learn to make the most of your assets—assets you
never knew you had. Develop a whole new
lease on life—and enjoy the NEW YOU!

Books by Linda A. Clark

STAY YOUNG LONGER
How to Add Years of Enjoyment to Your Life

GET WELL NATURALLY
Nature's Way to Health

SECRETS OF HEALTH AND BEAUTY
How to Make Yourself Over

SECRETS
OF HEALTH
AND BEAUTY

How to Make Yourself Over

by
LINDA A. CLARK, M.A.

 PYRAMID BOOKS • NEW YORK

To my mother, Mabelle,
who stood by with patience
and my daughters, Joan and Karen, who contributed
encouragement while I wrote this book

SECRETS OF HEALTH AND BEAUTY

A PYRAMID BOOK
Published by arrangement with The Devin-Adair Company

Seventh printing, February, 1974

PYRAMID BOOKS are published by Pyramid Communications, Inc.
Its trademarks, consisting of the word "Pyramid" and the portrayal
of a pyramid, are registered in the United States Patent Office.

Pyramid Communications, Inc.,
919 Third Avenue, New York, N.Y. 10022, U.S.A.

Contents

Foreword

In SECRETS OF HEALTH AND BEAUTY Linda Clark
gives us the key to radiant good looks and buoyant health.
And she does it in a new, exciting way . . . via herbs,
proteins, do-it-yourself cosmetics and easy-to-follow guidelines to sound nutrition.

This is a book to keep close at hand for constant re-
reading and reference. In it there is a regimen especially
meant for you and you will be rewarded many times over
when you find your own secrets of health and beauty and
put them to work.

Jheri Redding, M.S. Research Chemist in Cosmetics
Santa Barbara, California

Foreword

Linda Clark's devotion to a way of life dictated by natural rather than synthetic techniques, shines through the pages of this book. It is destined to reach and influence a much wider public, I believe, than her two earlier books, both of which have sold well in hard cover and paperback.

Especially interesting is Linda's own story, told here for the first time, of a sickly childhood and youth and of her discovery of the magic of sound nutrition. She is radiant proof of how well that discovery worked.

In SECRETS OF HEALTH AND BEAUTY she again proves her skill as a reporter in the nutritional and cosmetic fields. She presents her valuable findings simply and clearly and it is my personal wish that many thousands will share her discoveries and benefit by them.

Alan H. Nittler, M.D.

Santa Cruz, California

Preface: How This Book Can Help You

No matter what your age, sex, appearance, or health problem, it *is* possible to look better and feel better. Furthermore, it is never too late to begin.

Scientists state that your body completely rebuilds itself every seven years. Meanwhile, a continuous renewal process is taking place. Most cells need certain substances for this renewal process. If you learn what these substances are and how to use them, you can help to bring about almost unbelievable results in a surprisingly short time.

One example: if your skin is wrinkling, shriveling or dry, by following certain steps for rebuilding it both from the inside and from the outside of your body, your skin can acquire a sheen and become smoother. Many people who have used this method have improved an almost hopeless skin and are now proud of a beautiful complexion which brings them compliments wherever they go.

Many other benefits are also possible:

If your hair resembles dried straw, is lacklustre and anything but the crowning glory it was meant to be, you can turn it into a beautiful, glossy mane of which you can be proud.

If you are constantly fighting the battle of the bulge, there are unique, safe, and simple methods whereby you may attain a slim figure for life without hunger, weakness, looking haggard or wan.

If you are always tired, and are depending on such crutches to keep you going as pep pills, aspirin, coffee by the bucket, alcohol and tobacco, tranquilizers and sleeping pills, you can change all that, too. You can gain vibrant energy, and look as vital as you feel. Life, instead of being a drag, can be fun.

These are not idle promises. Many men and women have already reached these goals. Others are working toward them every day. The secrets of how to do it yourself, at home, appear in this book. But don't delude yourself that you can skip through the book, pick up one or more secrets, and succeed. You cannot. You must follow a complete, regular plan. Such a plan may even turn out to be a new way of life.

You will find all of the information you need for success in the pages which follow. I think you will find that the rewards of this approach to beauty, good looks, and good health will prove to be one of the best things to happen in your life.

The sooner you start, the sooner you will get results. The results can be permanent.

So let's begin, now, to make yourself over!

The information in this book is not intended as prescribing. As a reporter, I report only the findings of others. The information should be used in cooperation with a doctor who understands nutritional therapy. If this is impossible, you may use the information yourself, which is your constitutional right, since the substances discussed are foods, not drugs. The author and the publisher assume no responsibility.

PART I

HEALTH—THE FOUNDATION FOR BEAUTY

1 You Can Be More Beautiful

Must you deteriorate with age? Some people don't. This is not necessarily due to accident or luck. Nine times out of ten it is due to a planned program. Such a program can work even for people who have already deteriorated. They learn how to reverse the process, to look younger and more attractive.

Everyone wants to be more attractive. Women are not the only ones interested in their looks. Watch the average man, if you can catch him unaware, as he passes a mirror. He can't resist a glance at himself (unless he is afraid of the image he knows will be there). Usually, looking closely in his shaving mirror, he examines the pores of his skin, looks anxiously for approaching signs of baldness, or smiles at himself to determine what kind of impression he is going to make on the next attractive woman he meets.

Women, of course, preen too, except those who have lost their good looks and avoid a mirror. Fortunately, they can help to reverse their deterioration so that they can face themselves once more with pleasure. This is important to a woman who considers her appearance her life-line.

So, male or female, the dual business of how you feel and how you look is a major concern. The good news this book brings to you is that you can do something about it.

Good looks and good health are not necessarily a youngster's birthright. I know of an eight-year-old girl who was prematurely gray, with a withered skin, and looked as if she were in her seventies. By giving her certain substances, her hair turned brown, her skin became youthful, and she looked the age she was: eight instead of seventy. Aging can begin at any age. The magic which produced her improvement is known as nutrition. It can work in varying degrees for anyone.

WHERE TO BEGIN

You cannot look well unless you feel well. Most women try to camouflage their fading beauty with make-up, but the camouflage becomes less and less convincing. This is because they are going about it in the wrong way.

You must build a house before you paint it. Similarly, you must build your good looks permanently from the inside out. Working from the inside as the first step before decorating, you can reactivate body organs, glands, tissues, cells, and blood stream, which feed and control your appearance as well as your health. New exciting information contained in this book shows you how to rebuild or regenerate your skin and hair by using safe, effective nutritional substances on the inside of your body, at the same time applying them on the outside of your body. Using both methods simultaneously, you can get faster results than by either method alone.

Certain nutritional substances have been found to help rebuild cells. To get these nutrients on the inside of your body, you swallow them in the form of certain foods or food concentrates. To put them to work on the outside, you rub them on your skin or into your hair. This is a new, exciting concept.

Your body is constantly changing, trying to maintain, repair, and rebuild itself. Yet most people don't give it much help. By supplying the necessary reconstruction materials, you can help to perpetuate good health and good looks, and prevent, or help reverse, deterioration.

Dr. Melvin E. Page of the Page Biochemical Foundation in St. Petersburg, Florida, through research and wide experience, has found dramatic changes taking place once the body is chemically balanced. He finds in thousands of patients that the chemical imbalance is usually a result of improper diet, hastening the process of degeneration of health and appearance. After all, the outside of your body is but a mirror of its inner conditions.

One woman who uses this method of inside-outside nutritional approach to health and beauty is Gianna d'Angelo, the Metropolitan Opera soprano. She admits that she loves to eat, but tries to concentrate on fresh fruits and vegetables. In addition, she uses many of these same foods on her face.

For instance, she makes a mask of yogurt mixed with

organically raised strawberries (free from chemicals and sprays). Or she may add bananas or peaches, smoothing all ingredients in a blender before applying them as a cosmetic mask. She also combines yogurt with cucumber or herbs in the same manner. She leaves the mask on for 30 minutes and claims it does wonders for her dry skin.

Many other celebrities have learned the value of this twin-nutritional method. I have interviewed international beauty consultants and learned the secrets they teach stage, screen and television stars to acquire and protect their beauty and good looks by this technique. The list includes men, too. Those who use this fascinating and safe approach to health and beauty are so delighted with the results that they would not use any other. They are living proof that it works!

Just why does the inside-outside technique work? For explanation, let me tell you my own story.

2 Fads or Facts?

If anyone had told me years ago that I could regain my own health, I would not have believed it. Many people learn the hard way and I am one of them. However, I did regain it and I now know that others can do it, too. As I was learning, there were a few writers who had already established guideposts along the pathway to health, but because I am the "I'm from Missouri!" type, I had to find my own way and learn for myself that achieving better health is possible, once you know how. In this book I am going to show you this easy, workable method of improving your health, too, no matter what is wrong with you. As your health improves, so will your appearance.

It all started when I was born a sickly child. Owing to low resistance, I contracted everything that came along, from infant disturbances to all known childhood diseases. Although I was surrounded with loving relatives, had good medical care and plentiful food, I went downhill instead of up. It was not always continuous. I experienced some relatively good weeks, months, even years, but as a frail, delicate child, the trend was downward until, at the age of seven, I contracted a serious disease which lasted for months. The doctors did not expect me to live. In fact, the local weekly newspaper in our small town, not wanting to be laggard in reporting the news, accepted the medical verdict literally and printed my death notice ahead of time. (They had to retract it in the next issue.)

By some miracle, I got out of bed, finally on my feet, and made a slow recovery. However, the disease had left its mark and I was never able to keep up with other children. I always had to "watch my health." I managed to hold together long enough to finish college, marry, and produce two daughters. Then I began to backslide again.

This became apparent after our family had moved from a small college town to the New York City area. I suddenly realized that I was beginning to feel worse and worse. I could not walk up a flight of subway steps comfortably. My energy was waning and it was all I could do to complete my household chores.

I sought the help of several doctors—some specialists, some general physicians, all of whom agreed that I was suffering from at least five serious ailments or diseases. They recommended various drugs but I could see that they were not optimistic. None of these diseases was malignant, fortunately, but the doctors still considered me a pretty hopeless case. My determination came to my rescue, and before resigning myself to the doctor's verdict I decided there must be help elsewhere.

As early as junior high school I had been fascinated by "diet." In high school I had read every word I could find on the subject. In college I took every available course on nutrition. In those days little was known about the subject. Even so, when I applied to myself what little I learned, I found it always made me feel better. Later, when my two daughters were born, I practiced what I had learned on them.

For example, the children were not allowed refined sugar in any form. They were blissfully unaware of "sweets" until they attended an Easter egg hunt and ate their first candy Easter egg. To them this was like opening

Pandora's box. Nevertheless, I relentlessly pursued my nutritional convictions for the children, usually ignoring them for myself. They were becoming healthier and healthier while I was becoming sicklier and sicklier.

It did not occur to me that nutrition (or the lack of it) could have any connection with my own second siege of poor health. (I later learned it was even the cause of my original childhood problems.) Meanwhile, nutrition was definitely helping my children's health. As proof, one of my daughters, now a mother herself, recently told me, "I don't know what remedies to use if one of my children has a health upset. We did not need them or learn about them (aspirin, drugs, etc.) when we were growing up because we were almost never sick."

Meanwhile, poor health was upon me a second time, and I still did not recognize the cause.

My husband, who had been born a semi-invalid, and had also been plagued with continuing health problems, had already learned that the medical use of drugs was not the final solution for him. It had patched him up from time to time, but it didn't remove the cause of his poor health or prevent further illnesses. So he, too, was always on the lookout for some other means of help.

One day he came home with a book describing the effect of nutrition on health. He began to read it aloud to me while I was cooking or working in the kitchen. It mentioned vitamins, minerals, and such foods as blackstrap molasses, wheat germ, and brewers yeast. The book, by a college-trained writer, stated that surprising improvements had occurred for many people who used such foods. I was skeptical, having read warnings in magazines and heard radio and television broadcasts against such "health foods." According to these sources, they were mere "fads" and people who used them were "faddists." Those who promoted them were considered "quacks." Since I was unconsciously protecting my status, I did not want to be considered a faddist. So I paid no attention to the book.

Weeks later I turned on the radio to hear another side of the story: a health commentator was telling about case after case of poor health which had responded to "good nutrition." This rang a mental bell back to my school-day dietary studies, and I began to follow the program. The commentator cited cases from professional journals to back up his statements and even interviewed a few doctors on his program who seemed to agree with what he was telling the public. Later he mentioned and praised the book my husband had tried to read to me, and which I had rejected. Maybe, I thought, there is something to it after all.

So I began to read it for myself. I reasoned that since my health was already so poor, I had nothing to lose; perhaps it was worth a try. Making up my mind that I would not flinch if my friends called me a faddist, I decided to experiment and see what happened, to prove for myself whether such information was a fad or a fact.

3 Facts Win

Before I began my experiment I had the sympathy of my family, as well as that of my friends and neighbors, both because of my miserable health and because of the dire verdicts of the doctors. At first I told no one outside the family that I was trying out these new foods and nutrients. My family ate what I cooked (fortunately they considered me a good cook) so they were unwittingly sharing my experiment with me. They didn't complain about the new foods because I disguised them as much as possible and said nothing.

Gradually, results began to appear. Some days I began to feel better. On other days I felt the same old way. As I look back, it was similar to the add-a-pearl necklaces so popular many years ago. One good day was added now and then. Soon the good days were definitely increasing, the poor ones decreasing.

After years of health degeneration it is not surprising that improvement does not occur overnight. Many people expect instant relief through nutrition because drugs can give a temporary relief, say from a headache or insomnia. But though fine for emergency treatment, used as a way of life, drugs usually merely mask a condition, do not remove it. For example, aspirin stops the pain of a headache but does not remove the cause. Nutrition, on the other hand, rebuilds health. This takes time.

Finally it became undeniably clear that I was improving. I began to walk up stairs again with more ease. Energy was returning so that I could do my housework with less effort. Friends began to notice the difference and my own family found that I was less fragile and had more endurance. They, too, were feeling more energetic and all of us had noticed one thing in common: instead of our usual susceptibility to colds, we were having fewer and less serious ones.

In less than a year I was feeling, and apparently looking, like a different person. One friend tells me that she wished she had a before-and-after picture, because people to whom she tried to explain what had happened to me did not believe it.

Then I made a big mistake. It seemed so miraculous that instead of dragging through a normal day's activities, I was now surging with new vitality and energy, and I wanted to tell everyone about it. Unfortunately I tried. To my disappointment no one, outside of my family and a few close friends, was interested. They couldn't care less. They looked bored when I mentioned the subject. They, too, had read and heard the warnings about "health foods," and concluded that I had turned into a "faddist." If I brought up the subject at a party, which I often did, there was a strained silence before someone hurriedly changed the subject. My husband, who was now also convinced that nutrition was helping him as well as me, had the same experience with his business associates. It was clear that we were beginning to be considered "health nuts."

The harder we tried to explain, the worse the situation became. Many of our friends were suffering from one or more ailments, but they would not listen when we encouraged them at least to try nutrition. We finally realized that you cannot convert anyone to a different religion, politics, or a way of eating unless that person learns the facts for himself and wants to be converted. Many people have become nutrition-conscious only after coming to the end of their rope (as I did); or become frightened about the future of their health, having tried everything else without success. But you can't push most people. You can't shove them. You can't hurry them. They have to learn the facts for themselves, usually from reading, not from the advice of overanxious friends or relatives.

Even though I had experienced dramatic improvement, and my family were also showing proportionate improvement (less dramatic, since their health had not been as poor as mine), I felt completely frustrated because no one would believe that nutrition was responsible.

I decided to look for proof which would be convincing. Then I remembered the doctors and their original diagnoses. I had been feeling so well I had almost forgotten them. Now I decided to find out what their reaction was to my new feelings of well-being.

I returned to them, one by one, being particularly careful not to tell them at first what I had been doing. One by one, they re-examined me, compared my condition with the original diagnosis, and each one independently announced that *every disturbance which he had originally discovered had now been completely reversed!* There could be no excuse of mistaken diagnosis because they had all been in agreement.

They not only were surprised, they were curious. They asked me what I had been doing. Two general practitioners who lived in the same suburban town as I were particularly eager to know what had happened, and eventually I told them. But that is another story, to come later.

Formerly, I would have shouted this medical reprieve, this wonderful news from the housetops! But now I had learned my lesson. I knew the announcement, so overwhelming to me, would be shrugged off by others. I needed still more proof. And I needed it in writing, with statements from many others in addition to mine, before I could help to break through the barrier of nonbelief. I decided to look for it.

With an interest in research, nutrition, and degrees from two universities in a professional field, I had the necessary educational tools to acquire more learning. So I rolled up my sleeves, approached the largest medical library in New York City and went to work. For ten years I searched and researched for every shred of information I could find on the relationship between health and nutrition. What I learned I put in book form. The book is called *Stay Young Longer** and in it appear the findings of hundreds

---

* New York: Devin-Adair Company, 1961. Paperback edition—New York: Pyramid Books, 1968.

of scientists, experts, physicians—all testifying to the truth of this relationship.

The information was not easy to find. It often seemed as if it were deliberately being hidden from public view. I learned that nutrition was not even being taught to medical students, who, of all people, should know everything possible about health. The book contains indisputable proof and is, to my knowledge, the first nutrition book for the lay or average reader, complete with documentation from hundreds of professional and medical journals. Since I was reporting what scientists had learned about this subject, I avoided any statement which did not have documentation. Up to this time, anyone who had dared say these things was instantly labeled a "quack." Readers tell me *Stay Young Longer* has become a "bible" for those who are searching for health. It has also sufficiently impressed those in academic circles that it is being used as a textbook in four universities.

Most important, *Stay Young Longer* contains proof that nutrition *has* helped others as well as me.

Later I wrote a second book, *Get Well Naturally,** a sequel to the first. I listed many common diseases and showed what specific natural and nutritional treatments could be used for specific diseases. I also explained the mystery of why this information is being kept from the public. Documentation of proof is included.

I was listening recently to a discussion at a party attended by a number of "beautiful people." The women were dressed in the latest styles, had fresh hair-dos and carefully applied make-up. Suddenly a newcomer arrived. She came in like a fresh breeze. Her hair was clean and bouncy; she wore little make-up; her eyes danced. Every man—and woman—turned to look and admire this attractive, energetic newcomer. She did not stay long, but while she did, she was the center of attention.

Later some of the guests were trying to analyze why she captured attention. She was not as beautifully coiffed, made up, or as well dressed as the others. Finally someone said, "I've got it. It's her health and vitality. It shows in her hair, skin, eyes, figure—even in the way she walks."

I know now that nutrition is one of the keys which unlock the door to such abundant vitality.

---

* New York: Devin-Adair Company, 1965; Arc Book paperback, 1968.

I am going to tell you why the nutritional approach works successfully. Once you understand it you can apply it to your health and appearance, too.

4   How It Works

Before you start to improve your health, which will be almost immediately reflected in your improved appearance, it will make more sense to you if you understand what has caused your present state of health.

You are a law unto yourself. No one else has the same fingerprints or the same exact characteristics. No one else really understands you as well as you do (or could, if you tried diligently).

STUDY YOURSELF

One university professor learned the value of studying himself. Whenever he did not feel well, he began to analyze what he had eaten or drunk the day before. When he located the culprit he asked his wife not to serve it to him again. This may be an extreme approach, but it worked for that professor. He lived to be a hale and hearty ninety-one years old.

Not long ago, following one of my lectures, a woman came up to me and said, "I do not live near a doctor who understands nutritional therapy. Where can I go for advice?"

I answered, "Study yourself."

She brightened. "That is exactly what I did. I went to twenty-five different doctors seeking a diagnosis for my problem and I received twenty-five different diagnoses. I finally decided to study myself. I discovered my trouble and I'm correcting it. But," (and she looked a little dubious), "I thought you weren't supposed to diagnose yourself."

Some people cannot diagnose themselves. Obviously, if you need a helping hand, this is what physicians are for. However, if you cannot find acceptable help, it is certainly worth a try to do it yourself, and it is better than doing nothing at all. After all, it is your body.

A medical journal, read by most physicians in the United States, recently announced that two German doctors have discovered, as a result of reading and study, that one-third of their patients made correct diagnoses of their own ailments before seeking medical opinion. The better educated the patient, the more accurate the diagnosis. Those with high school or college education were found to be 62 per cent correct in their self-diagnosis.

WHAT CAUSES MOST POOR HEALTH?

Scientists have analyzed the human body and found that it is composed of 60 or more elements. (Some investigators believe there may be as many as 103.) Whatever the number, these elements are apparently necessary to maintain health of cells, glands, and organs. If any of these elements is missing from your body, trouble develops. The trouble may not show up next week or next month, but sooner or later the deficiency is bound to take its toll. H. W. Holderby, M.D., states that the body needs all 60 of these elements; 30 or 15 will not do the job. All 60 are necessary.

Technically we should all be born with a full supply of these health-giving elements, but such is not always the case. For instance, several top-flight university scientists, in trying to discover the cause of the increasing number of birth defects, learned that malformed babies did not receive some of these nutrients, necessary for perfect development, during pregnancy. One study pinpointed again and again the fact that certain defects appeared with clocklike regularity when the fetus was deprived of a single nutrient at a specific time during the growth period. For instance, a cleft palate occurred when one certain nutrient was unavailable to the baby during one of the early weeks of pregnancy.*

* Howard A. Hilleman, M.D., "Congenital Deformity," *Journal of Applied Nutrition*, Vol. XII, No. 4, 1959.

Even the thalidomide disasters were later found to prove this point. The malformations from this drug were eventually traced, not so much to the drug itself, but to the lack of a vitamin B-2, which, if it had been supplied through the mother's diet, would have protected the baby from birth defects. This information has been conclusively proved with many animals and some people.

Other defects, including weak heart, poor vision and hearing, and subnormal gland activity, have now been traced to such depletion during pregnancy.

The deficiency principle follows the same pattern from birth throughout adulthood. Even though a person may be born with an adequate supply of nutrients, if they are not constantly replaced as fast as they are being used up by the body, the supply will eventually dwindle. Glands, organs, and cells, dependent on those nutrients for efficient operation, will be forced to feed upon the body itself (as in total fasting when no food is being supplied) in order to survive.

Let's look at calcium as an example. If you are not taking enough in your diet, the body will steal it from the areas in your body where it is normally stored: bones and teeth. Thus a breakdown will sooner or later take place wherever this theft has occurred. Irritability, arthritis, osteoporosis of the bones, or tooth decay may develop. And remember, calcium is just one element. If there are 59 others in short supply, many deficiencies can eventually create havoc in your body. Such disturbances are called deficiency or degenerative diseases.

In light of this information, my own case now became clear to me. When I questioned my mother, she admitted that before I was born her diet had become depleted prior to, and during, her pregnancy. She even worried, she said, for fear the excruciating leg cramps from which she was suffering beforehand would appear during delivery. This was a complete giveaway, because we know today that such leg cramps are due to a calcium deficiency. When calcium is supplied, this type of leg cramps disappears.

So I started life as a nutritional cripple and became a target for every childhood disease. Whereas other children with a stronger inheritance might have resisted these diseases entirely, or at least suffered only a mild case, I had a serious case of everything. Later, due to ignorance, I failed to give myself an adequate supply of all the nutrients. The toll was exacted from my glands, organs, and cells, and my "five degenerative diseases" finally developed.

Once understood, this idea is so simple, we wonder why we never thought of it before. Deficiency diseases often take one form in one person, another in another. They usually strike in the weakest spot. But the underlying cause is the same: the inadequate supply of construction or repair materials. Such diseases may include heart ailments, arthritis, fatigue, insomnia, anemia, and a host of others. Even infectious diseases, caused by a germ or virus, can be more serious if protective elements are lacking and body resistance is correspondingly lowered. In support of this, at Rockefeller Institute, studies with mice showed that though good nutrition did not change the bacterial infections in the body, it strengthened the host's resistance to the germs.

It is also true that psychological and environmental problems can play their part.

CAN POOR HEALTH BE REVERSED?

If you do supply the missing or depleted nutrients, will you reverse poor health? Yes. This is the whole concept of nutrition: by giving the body the necessary repair materials, it can begin to repair itself. If provided prior to illness it can prevent it. If given afterward, health is usually improved.

Is there proof that this does happen? Yes. Radioactive tracers have been used to note what happens when various substances are given to the body. For example, if liver is supplied it makes a bee-line for the liver to start its work there. If a food such as heart or kidney is supplied, the same thing happens. If all of the substances are mixed together, the wonderful mechanism of the body sorts them out and delivers each substance to the right place: liver to liver, heart to heart, kidney to kidney, and so on. As each nutrient necessary for the health and survival of each organ and gland is supplied, all are picked up and put to work to start the repair process. Sooner or later the glands and organs are humming once more as the body machinery begins to run more normally.

This explains how I and thousands of others have regained health through nutrition. Countless examples have come to light. Dr. Lowell Langstroth found as early as 1929 that in 500 of his patients the more protective foods his patients ate, the fewer degenerative diseases they acquired. By placing 274 of his patients suffering from degenerative conditions, such as heart disease, indigestion, and migraine headaches, on a diet containing 60 per cent of the necessary nutrients, 33 of his patients obtained complete relief; 56 per cent showed slight to marked improvement.

I have already warned that improvement usually does not take place overnight. The greater the depletion, or the longer the deficiencies have existed, the longer the recovery time. Some experts go so far as to state that once the body has been subjected to the stress of disease, it may always carry with it the "scar" of that illness, resulting in over-sensitivity. Thus, when health has been achieved for such an individual, he or she may have to stick to the new nutritional program forever in order to prevent backsliding.

There are some people, however, who seem to defy all of these rules. They eat anything and everything, and still remain healthy! It is maddening to the rest of us who try so hard to follow the correct nutritional procedure (and pay the piper when we don't, with a minor upset such as indigestion or fatigue) only to watch others consistently break all the rules and apparently thrive! It took me some time to find out why.

I watched a family of three. Two brothers and one sister reached the respective ages of seventy-nine, eighty-nine, and ninety-nine. For their ages they were in remarkable health. Their hair showed very little gray; they still had their own teeth; they were alert and active. Yet they never took a vitamin or mineral, nor ate a balanced diet. They subsisted on what I call "junk"; foodless foods which fill up the stomach but lack the protective elements necessary for constant body repair.

After questioning them at length I learned that their parents had lived on a farm. They had eaten a nutritious, farm-fresh diet, full of protective nutrients. They also had plenty of exercise, pure water and air, and were perfect specimens of health. In turn, they bequeathed a good glandular system (the machinery which helps run the body) to their children, who also lived, and ate the same nutritious food, on the farm for many years. So this heritage protected these "children" who were seventy-nine, eighty-nine, and ninety-nine far longer into adulthood than people like me who had started life with a nutritional deficit.

A man who understands this inherited-gland principle was recently marveling at an elderly woman who runs a small restaurant. She does all the cooking herself, works long hours, sleeps little, and exhibits abundant energy. She, too, hails from hardy stock and is a living example of a wholesome diet. The man, at least twenty years younger, sighed enviously and said to her, "Mary, how I wish I had your glands!"

This sequence of inheritance-plus-good-nourishment occurs in animals. One monumental study of cats showed that the poor effects of nutrition did not show up in the first generation at all. But in the second generation, ailments similar to those suffered by humans made their appearance. Health became still worse during the third generation, and by the time the fourth generation arrived the health problems had become practically hopeless.

Plants also reflect good or poor inheritance. So it is not surprising that people do too. Someone has remarked, "One of the best ways to have good health is to pick the right parents." Inheritance is important, but what most people do not realize is that their parents' health was influenced by *their* diet. So proper nourishment, plus good health inheritance, is important.

Even those who escape—for a while—have a day of reckoning. I finally witnessed it in every one of those three "children" who had reached seventy-nine, eighty-nine, and ninety-nine. One day the younger one collapsed. On being rushed to the hospital he was found to have everything wrong with him: his heart, liver, kidneys had apparently collapsed simultaneously. His body, though it had appeared fairly normal on the outside, on the inside gave the impression of a house riddled by termites. He died. Shortly afterward, one by one, the others followed the exact pattern. The lack of repair materials had finally caught up with them. Such complete breakdowns could have been prevented.

HOW TO SUCCEED

Most of us take our bodies for granted. We let our health and our appearance operate on a hit-or-miss principle. But this need not be. You can learn to control the way you feel and the way you look by cooperating with the master plan of self-renewal.

As one scientist explains it, "Your body needs certain

nutrients for energy, growth, and repair. When you take in food it goes through the process of digestion, which breaks down proteins, starches, vitamins, and minerals for assimilation. During digestion, fats are also split into their finer parts. And as the digested material passes over the surface lining of the small intestine, it is absorbed into the blood. In this way nourishment reaches all the cells of your body."

Herein lies the first clue to success.

When you understand what nutrients to choose to be delivered to your cells and tissues for their repair, then you become the captain of your ship, instead of leaving it to chance. You can deliberately put these elements to work to rebuild your body, and once attained by the same process, maintain good health indefinitely. You can learn to prevent the many illnesses which plague those who do not understand this principle. Such knowledge is a weapon against unnecessary aging and deterioration. In years past, monarchs would have paid a king's ransom for it. Today the secrets are available to you, as presented here. The only requirement is that you learn them and apply them. The potential is almost staggering in its possibilities. Stop and consider: by applying this knowledge you can largely control the way you feel and the way you look the rest of your life.

Before you begin, a preliminary step is necessary for most people in order to ensure speedier results. This first important step in your rehabilitation program is discussed in the next chapter.

5 Get Rid of Those Poisons

To be sure that your body, skin, and hair can take full advantage of the necessary repair materials, you need to assimilate them efficiently. If you are choked with poisons, as most people are, your progress will be considerably slowed. If, on the other hand, you do a little sensible housecleaning, you should make faster progress and get observable results perhaps within a few days; certainly within a few weeks.

You may have been unaware that your body is clogged with poisons. Yet this is true of most people in civilized countries today. Alan H. Nittler, M.D., an expert in this field, says: "When abnormal substances which do not belong there, get into the body, they must be neutralized and expelled. These substances may be poisons, drugs, preservatives, artificial sweeteners (particularly the calcium and sodium cyclamates), softeners, alkalizers, acidifiers, hormones, dyes, antioxidants, hydrogenators, etc. ad infinitum. There are over 2,500 different chemicals allowed in our foods one way or another (you will find many of them by reading labels on the food you buy, though many are often unlisted and invisible).

"In all, there are about 8,000 different chemicals in our total environment which we can breathe, drink, eat or touch. Some are potent poisons, others are less active; but all are abnormal to the human body and must be neutralized or excreted, or else disease, even death, can result."

How can you get rid of these substances which accumulate in the body? A detoxifying diet can cleanse and remove much debris from organs, glands, tissues, and blood stream. It can be particularly helpful in cleansing the walls of the small intestine, which become encrusted with undigested food and form a barrier to the absorption of important nutrients into the blood stream. But the type of detoxification diet must be chosen with great care. Otherwise more harm than benefit may occur.

FASTING CAN BE DANGEROUS

One way to start a heated argument is to state unequivocally that people should or should not fast. I know, because I have started them. The trouble is that the word "fast" means different things to different people. There are many varieties: juice fasts, fruit fasts, raw-food fasts, even Lenten fasts which eliminate only one type of food, such as sweets or meat. The most common concept, however, is a total fast, meaning that a person drinks only water and eats no food at all. This type of fasting is now considered dangerous by investigators who have studied its effects.

It is true that total fasting was at one time highly recommended. It has even been mentioned in the Bible. But many changes have taken place in our universe since then. The world is now being gradually contaminated with pollutants of all kinds, and our bodies are soaking them up. One of these is insecticides. DDT is applied directly to plants and growing food. It also settles on the soil which remains contaminated for years. Insecticides can thus become embedded or built into the foods via the soil and cannot be washed off. Still worse, as a result of spraying in some areas, DDT drifts on wind currents to other uncontaminated areas, where it drops to earth. As a result, insecticides are turning up all over the globe.

A man, known as the "Lettuce King of America," talked with me about this problem. He has gained this title because he raises and ships the largest supply of lettuce in the United States. I was explaining my concern over the insecticide-treated lettuce most Americans are eating today. He was concerned, too, but for a different reason. He said, "I wish we had never started to use insecticides. Each year we have to use more and more because the bugs are becoming more and more resistant to them."

Meanwhile we, the people, are taking more and more of this poison into our bodies, where it is stored in the fatty tissues and the liver. This gradual accumulation can lead to serious complications, and plays havoc with health and appearance.

There are hazardous results from sudden, intense exposure to such poisons. A dear friend, an internationally known agricultural scientist and statesman, argued the pros and cons of insecticides with me for many years. He upheld their use because they contributed, he said, to a greater yield of food. I claimed, on the other hand, that natural, safe insect controls were preferable because they didn't poison the people as well as the bugs. (Insecticides kill bugs by paralyzing their nervous systems.)

One day I learned that my friend was critically ill. His illness seemed to be a traveling form of nerve paralysis and it was relentlessly creeping from one part of his body to another. Outstanding physicians and hospitals in two countries gave the illness a fancy name, but they were baffled by it and helpless to treat it.

I received a letter from my friend, who wrote: "This is the hardest admission of my life. I have always supported insecticides. Now I believe they are the cause of my trouble. I was in perfect health until the day I was handling some special crop species which had just been heavily sprayed with DDT. As I look back on it, this was the beginning of my illness. It is true that insecticides may produce bigger crops, but you are right; it is a dangerous procedure."

This brilliant, internationally known scientist died of the same paralyzing symptoms which destroy bugs.

FASTING AND INSECTICIDES

I have told this story because there is a direct connection between fasting and insecticides. It is true that not everyone is contaminated suddenly with concentrated doses of these poisons. Many people accumulate them slowly, but surely, in small amounts derived from various sources, particularly from the foods they eat. DDT exists in some degree in nearly every person today. It has even been found in babies, before and after birth.

Should you begin a total fast, using only water and no food, your body is forced to feed upon itself in lieu of food. As the fatty tissues, where the insecticides are stored, begin to break down, the poisons are too rapidly released into the blood stream. They become your sole "nourishment." Thus you can poison yourself. For this reason, total fasting has caused illness, occasional death.

Yet insecticides are only one of the many poisons we are exposed to daily. Other poisons are stored in the body, too. When you fast you are providing your body with an undiluted menu of poisons.

One man who has advocated total fasting for years, both in lectures as well as in a book he has written, is still claiming that it is beneficial. He apparently does not realize that our world has changed in the last twenty years and that earlier rules no longer apply. I have not seen him, but I have been told that he is a walking skeleton. His own health is threatened, yet he continues to "total fast," hoping for improvement. He is unaware that he is repeating a vicious cycle of poisoning and repoisoning himself.

On the other hand, I know of another health devotee, who also recommends fasting. He is in excellent health. His concept of a fast, however, is different. He recommends the use of fresh juices, and raw fruits and vegetables as cleansing mediums. By the intake of such foods, the poisons are released slowly, not suddenly. They are diluted so that the body can release and excrete them more safely. Furthermore, this man has screened his diet for years so that so far as possible he does not eat or drink any contaminated food. He uses only natural products, pure water, and foods which have been organically grown, thus uncontaminated by sprays and chemicals. Few of us are as discriminating about what we put into our bodies. In generations past everyone automatically ate such pure, wholesome food. Not so today. We must search for such hard-to-find food. Later I will make suggestions where to obtain it.

Before you start on any diet, it is wise to check with a nutritional physician. Since they are rare, it might be well to alert your family doctor to keep an eye on you while you diet. Most doctors were trained before the advent of insecticides and other pollutants and thus do not recognize the symptoms of such poisoning when they encounter them. They often shrug off such a disturbance as being due to "your imagination," or a "virus," or just "something going around." I have watched epidemics of illnesses carrying these dubious labels and noted that they often coincide with the release of certain heavily sprayed foods which have just reached the market.

In case you cannot find a professional who understands these problems to supervise your detoxifying diet, you can follow the suggestions of the following three doctors judiciously. If you learn what to expect, you should, like hundreds of others, come through with flying colors.

HOW TO START

Method I

Alan H. Nittler, M.D., whom I have previously mentioned, starts his patients on a three-day detoxification diet of fresh, organic carrot juice, or other freshly prepared raw vegetable juices. (You can buy a juicer and make your own.)

In case you are unable to find safe, organically raised carrots or other vegetables (those uncontaminated by chemicals and insecticide sprays), Dr. Nittler suggests two alternatives; a diet of well-washed, well-chewed grapes; or a diet of whole grapefruit and celery. Whatever your choice, additional vitamins are recommended throughout the diet.

Whichever juices or foods you choose, Dr. Nittler says that you may drink or eat them as often as you wish, whenever you are hungry. The hardest part of any diet is the first three days when your stomach is shrinking and demanding more food. After that you usually reach the I-don't-care stage.

After the three days, preferably of juices, Dr. Nittler places his patients on raw fruit and vegetables (plus vitamins) for up to three weeks. This is not as hard as it sounds and the results are highly rewarding. Dr. Nittler states that his patients soon look and feel more alert, have a spring in their step, sleep better, and have more energy.

I recall a friend who, many years ago, remained on this type of raw-food diet prescribed by her doctor, for an extended time. His purpose for the diet was to eliminate a physical disturbance which was traced to body toxins. The surprising result, however, was the woman's appearance. Everyone who knew her exclaimed over it. She looked fresh, more attractive and younger as her diet advanced. She actually appeared to be rejuvenated. This was no doubt due to the effect of cleansing the poisons from her body.

Such a raw-food diet can be delicious. Vegetables can be used in salads with a dressing of cold-pressed oils, apple cider vinegar or lemon juice; seasoned with sea salt, which contains more minerals than regular salt, but tastes identical. Fruits can be made into salads, fruit cups, or eaten separately. The variations are endless and the diet truly satisfying.

After three weeks' time, Dr. Nittler gradually adds proteins to his patients' diet in order of ease of digestion: yogurt; then fish, fowl and lamb; finally veal and beef. He does not favor pork.

Method II

Kurt Donsbach, D.C., N.D., believes that the liver is usually in great need of detoxification. This makes sense because the liver is the organ which filters all poisons which enter your body. If it becomes clogged, it can no longer help your body efficiently to get rid of poisons. The net result may be a general feeling of sluggishness, or one or more body disturbances. Dr. Donsbach has found that his patients have had excellent success with the following liver-detoxifying diet. He says, "It is a comparatively simple diet, easy to follow, and takes only three days."

He has been besieged with requests for printed copies of the diet. Here it is:

Begin with a liquid fast consisting of the following:
1st day: Juice of a dozen medium-sized lemons mixed with sufficient honey in 2 quarts of water to make a palatable drink (the honey should be natural, unrefined, unsprayed). Juice sufficient raw beet tops and roots to make 2 fluid ounces.
2nd day: Repeat lemon, honey, and water mixture, but juice 4 fluid ounces of beet juice.
3rd day: Repeat lemon, honey, and water mixture, but add 6 fluid ounces of beets.

"Come off this program gently," advises Dr. Donsbach, "adding other juices as you desire, but specifically deleting from your diet citrus juice of any kind. It is also recommended that you abstain from eating any white sugar or white flour product of any kind, and avoid drinking pasteurized milk or eating pasteurized dairy products."

He concludes, "You will find that the general feeling of well-being which follows such a program will encourage you to repeat this diet at least once every month or six weeks to give your liver a chance to return to normal."

Method III

I am particularly impressed with a detoxifying diet formulated by Stanley A. Burroughs, a teacher of natural health. Mr. Burroughs calls this diet the "Master Cleanser." He says it can accomplish the following:

—Dissolve and eliminate toxins and waste anywhere in the body.
—Give the digestive system a rest.
—Act as a purifier for glands, cells, and blood stream.
—Help weight loss of approximately a pound a day.
—Feed the body at the same time it is being cleansed.
—Help maintain youth and elasticity regardless of age.

This diet, too, is simple: combine the juice of one-half lemon (about 2 tablespoons) with 2 tablespoons of blackstrap molasses in an 8-ounce glass of medium-hot water. That is all there is to it.

According to Mr. Burroughs you can drink this mixture whenever you get hungry—from six to twelve times daily, as you wish. He suggests pure maple syrup or sorghum as alternatives to the molasses. We do know, however, that a blackstrap molasses analysis shows an extremely high level of minerals and vitamins.* Furthermore, since blackstrap is a natural laxative, constipation does not develop. If you are a diabetic or find the laxative effects of the blackstrap too great, Mr. Burroughs suggests reducing the amount of blackstrap to one tablespoon per glass.

Should you feel the need of more energy, from time to time while you are on this diet, you may cut up the whole lemon, skin, seeds and all, and liquefy it together with the water and blackstrap in your blender. The whole lemon is a rich source of bioflavonoids, better known as the vitamin C family or complex.

Mr. Burroughs suggests that you remain on this diet as long as possible up to ten days, and repeat it three or four times a year to prevent reaccumulation of waste products and toxins. People who have tried this diet become particularly enthusiastic about the compliments they receive on how well and young they look. Mr. Burroughs agrees that this high vitamin-mineral cleansing diet helps you to look and feel your best.

HOW DETOXIFICATION CAN IMPROVE YOUR APPEARANCE

One woman, an expert in nutrition, has led hundreds of people to better health and appearance. She herself is an excellent example. Her skin and hair are beautiful and her health radiant. She says this was not always so; she acquired both through proper nutrition, used inside and out. She firmly believes, however, that to achieve success, before you apply beautifying substance to the outside of your body, you must begin on the inside.

She says, "You cannot have a clear skin if your intestines are clogged with toxins and poisons, which leads to a toxic liver. Your skin reflects these conditions. It will not be clear, and brown spots (often called liver spots) on hands or face are merely a sign that poisons have piled up in the intestines and liver."

She has helped numerous clients to get rid of these horrid spots by the use of a certain natural formula. She says, "Don't watch the spots too closely. Take a colored picture of yourself, if you wish, then forget about them. Within

---

* See analysis in Linda Clark, *Stay Young Longer*.

three to six months you will notice they are fading or have faded."

This woman's detoxification formula is based upon research by Metchnikoff, the Russian scientist, who examined many men and women who had lived in the Balkans to the ripe age of 100 to 125. He found they all had one factor in common: they had drunk one quart of yogurt daily all their lives. The skin of these people was clear and beautiful. Yogurt, beside having other advantages, contains friendly bacilli which act as an intestinal cleanser. It has been used in Europe for centuries. Americans are just beginning to realize its benefits. Using the Metchnikoff discovery as a clue, the nutritionist has found an easier and more potent method which she has used herself and has recommended to hundreds of others. Here is her detoxification plan for beauty:

In connection with your regular diet, drink twice daily three tablespoons of liquid acidophilus plus one tablespoon of lactose (milk sugar) or whey, to an 8-ounce glass of water. Take one tablespoon desiccated liver (or 30 tablets) daily (all these products are available at health food stores) or eat fresh liver once a week to help regenerate your liver. This program is continued indefinitely.

She reports that people who use this method return in six months enthusiastically revealing a clearer skin, unclouded eye whites, and fading or faded brown spots. Her own peaches-and-cream complexion is visible proof that her method can be successful.

Another type of friendly bacillus has come to our attention. It is known as Lactobacillus bifidus. Recent European medical opinion (as presented in the *American Journal of Proctology*, Vol. 19, No. 5) reports that adding Bifidus in powder form to the diet helps the breakdown of food particles in the lower intestine, keeps harmful germs at bay, and destroys toxins resulting from waste accumulation in the colon.

Bifidus is being used by European physicians for liver regeneration, particularly in cases of hepatitis. It is easy to combine the Bifidus powder, which comes in a malt or whole milk base, with water for a delicious beverage. Since it serves as an excellent natural enzyme for internal cleansing it can be used as a long-range detoxification method alone. Physicians note that although some people report good results within two weeks, it may take up to 8 months of continuous use if no other detoxifying measures are used. In short, it is an easy, delicious, but longer method of detoxification. It is now available in the United States in many health stores.

NECESSARY PRECAUTIONS

There are certain precautions to observe in any food fast or detoxifying diet:

Do not be surprised if, at some time during the diet, you feel temporarily worse. This is a sign the poisons are being dislodged and distributed throughout your body before excretion, and is often called the "healing crisis." It gradually disappears in direct ratio to the disappearance of the poisons.

To speed the removal of the toxins, particularly if constipation is present, Dr. Nittler, and many other therapists, recommend enemas for a few days. Exercise, bathing, and deep breathing also help. Many doctors use large doses of vitamin C (ascorbic acid) to neutralize the poisons.

Coffee drinkers should taper off their coffee. A sudden cessation often causes headaches. One method is to drink half coffee-half decaffeinated coffee, gradually increasing the one and decreasing the other. Herb teas, available in health stores, are good substitutes. Many are delicious.

When you do return to solid food, begin gently. Choose easily digested foods; eat small amounts, and chew them until they reach the liquid state.

After your detoxification diet is completed, screen your food carefully. Avoid refined, processed, contaminated food, or food treated with additives of any kind. As someone has jokingly remarked, if you can't understand or pronounce the chemicals listed on those foods which are honestly labeled, don't buy the food! Patient label-reading in supermarkets and shopping at health-food stores can provide a safer diet. If your health-food store does not stock organically grown fruits and vegetables, they may be able to recommend a source. There is a partial list of national suppliers of organic foods in two magazines: *Organic Gardening and Farming* (Emmaus, Pennsylvania 18049) and *Natural Food and Farming* (P.O. Box 210, Atlanta, Texas 75551).

If possible, grow some of your own food. Even if you live on a city lot, tuck some lettuce, carrots, and beets among your flowers. The foliage is pretty and you can personally guarantee they are unsprayed.

Once your body is cleansed, in addition to choosing your food carefully, how else can you ensure yourself against a reaccumulation of toxins?

The next chapter contains, in my opinion, some of the most important, yet some of the most overlooked, information for good health and good looks I have ever found.

6   An Undiscovered Genie

In the helter-skelter times in which we are living, most people are not thoroughly digesting their food. Dr. E. Hugh Tuckey, of San Francisco, a member of a husband-and-wife team of doctors, now retired, says, "We have seen patients by the hundreds, who came into the office, and were living on a splendid, well-balanced diet, yet complaining of bloat, gas, constipation, often foul breath—the same conditions you would expect from people living on a poor diet.

"We found, after giving colonic irrigations, that waste substances were visible, in the view tube, of foods which had been eaten six or seven days earlier. This food had not been properly acidified, digested or broken down, and had begun to putrefy. Gas had begun to form, followed by characteristic belching.

"Such people would go to bed, not feeling too bad, only to wake up with a burning in their stomachs. Their natural assumption was that they were suffering from too much acid. They would get up and take bicarbonate of soda or a commercial antacid. This turned out to be the worst thing they could do! The reason: the symptoms of too little acid *are exactly the same as too much acid*. Thus, we found that these people were suffering from too little acid, rather than too much. When acid was given to them, instead of antacids, their symptoms cleared up."

This statement is hard for the American public to accept.

They are bombarded by radio and television commercials telling them to take this, that, or another brand of antacid. An antacid gives only temporary relief from the symptoms and actually can make the basic condition eventually worse.

Dr. Tuckey states, "The media of the stomach is acid and if it isn't acid, you are in trouble. Acid is necessary to break down proteins and minerals for digestion, as well as to destroy certain bacteria. If enough acid does not exist, the emptying time of the stomach is slowed down, the bacteria are not destroyed and food which was eaten yesterday or even several days before, is not digested. Often it remains in the stomach, where it begins to cause trouble. The type of digestion which takes place in the mouth has nothing to do with that which takes place in the stomach, and the two should not be confused."

The Doctors Tuckey spent thirty years of independent research with many hundreds of patients. They finally discovered the cause of, as well as the solution to, the problem of their many patients who complained of indigestion.

Dr. Tuckey says, "When these people would come into our office in the early years of our practice we would try to understand why they were suffering from these symptoms. We used various types of products with little success. Finally we turned our attention to hydrochloric acid. After trying liquid hydrochloric acid sipped through a glass tube, which had very little lasting effect on the patient, we discovered a tablet form of HCL (the chemical abbreviation for hydrochloric acid). We learned that it, too, didn't work very well unless it had pepsin in it. We finally arrived at the conclusion that a tablet which contains hydrochloric acid betaine plus pepsin (now available in health stores) did the best work of all. Some people had a deficiency of HCL. Some had no HCL at all. In either case, we found we could normalize the hydrochloric acid in their stomachs."

SOME GOOD RESULTS WITH HCL

Dr. Tuckey gives an example of how HCL can destroy one type of stomach bacteria which causes diarrhea. He says, "We had many patients who went to Mexico and came back with what is commonly called *Turista. Turista* is a violent type of diarrhea from which the victim suffers great discomfort and pain. There are some drugs and antibiotics usually given to counteract it but in spite of them, our laboratory analysis found that these *Turista* species of bacteria still remained in the intestines three or four years later.

"So we began giving our patients a bottle of hydrochloric acid tablets when they went to Mexico. My wife and I went there many times, too, and always took the HCL along the way. All of us were able to enjoy our Mexican vacations without succumbing either to the dreaded diarrhea or from any side effects of the HCL."

Many people are traveling worldwide these days. They are constantly warned against eating or drinking food or beverage in unsanctioned restaurants. Even so, a case of diarrhea may accidentally develop. In spite of the fact that the traveler may follow all the rules, drink bottled or boiled water, he may thoughtlessly brush his teeth with tap water and swallow bacteria which cause diarrhea.

A friend of mine picked up diarrhea from an unknown source in India. It persisted after she returned to the United States. It defied every antibiotic and all medical treatment. She became progressively weaker. Her weight dropped to a dangerous low. Finally, after endless laboratory analyses and treatments, one physician recommended hydrochloric acid for an indefinite time. She completely recovered.

A CHAIN REACTION

The investigations of Dr. Tuckey solved a few other riddles, too, which had been plaguing not only his patients but physicians as well.

He explains: "When we have a deficiency of hydrochloric, we begin to see other things happen. In all patients with either a deficiency, or complete lack of HCL, we always found a spastic pylorus (opening to the small intestine). We did not guess at this. We have demonstrated this clinically one hundred times out of one hundred! This spastic condition leads to incorrect emptying of the bile duct and the pancreatic duct. The liver normally secretes, and the gall bladder normally excretes two or three pints of bile daily.

"But if the pylorus or opening to the small intestine is in a state of spasm and does not empty properly, the normal amount of bile cannot empty into the small intestine. One of the properties of bile is that it is a bactericide. It destroys the alkaline bacteria which are not destroyed in the stomach. It also promotes peristalsis, that wormlike motion of the small intestine which leads to elimination. Without the proper amount of bile, a sluggish bowel or constipation results. Meanwhile the liver is engorged with bile which should be going into the small intestine. But that is not all.

"The pancreas has to help digest proteins, fats, and carbohydrates. Without sufficient HCL and bile, an extra burden is put on the pancreas; the head of the pancreas becomes enlarged; and in those people who develop chronic pancreatitis, the pancreas becomes hard and tender.

"The man or woman who has pancreatitis (or even hepatitis) can take all the liver formulas available, and diet assiduously, and it will bring no results. I have treated more people with pancreatitis than any one of my professional acquaintances, and with few exceptions we found a deficiency of hydrochloric acid.

"So the lack of hydrochloric acid has started a whole chain of difficulties: liver, gall bladder and pancreas involvement leading to indigestion; gas, belching, bloating, constipation; sometimes diarrhea and vomiting; inability to assimilate food (no matter how good the diet) and imperfect elimination."

This results in the encrustation or impaction of the small intestine as mentioned earlier.

MANY DISEASES RESPOND TO HCL

Stored toxins and putrefaction are a good beginning for many other ailments, as you will soon see. But there are other consequences of a shortage—or complete lack—of HCL. Dr. Tuckey was one of the first to discover the fact that minerals, as well as protein, could not be digested without sufficient HCL.

Dr. Tuckey adds, "Today, no doctor would make a diagnosis of pernicious anemia without first establishing the diagnosis of a deficiency of HCL in the stomach. Iron cannot be broken down and delivered to the red blood cells without acid.

"Furthermore, in all the years I practiced I never saw an arthritic patient, and I have treated them by the hundreds, who did not have a deficiency of hydrochloric acid as well as a deficiency of calcium. Calcium, too, needs acid for proper assimilation. When we produced a balance

in the hydrochloric acid and corrected the calcium deficiency, although the X-rays did not necessarily demonstrate
changes in the arthritic condition, we helped our patients
become, and remain, pain-free. We sent them back to
work.

"One ailment which often plagues people is pruritis ani,
or itching of the rectum. We find it occurring around the
holidays when people eat too many sweets, carbohydrates
or chocolate, etc. Generally, when we took those patients
off sweets the disturbance would clear up. But later we
learned that hydrochloric acid would clear up the condition once and for all.

"Halitosis is another condition which responds to HCL.
One of my favorite professors, who later died of cancer,
had been a vegetarian for thirty or forty years. He had
such a foul breath that you had to turn your back to him—
even at thirty paces. Usually those with halitosis will find
their bad breath will disappear very quickly when HCL is
normalized in the stomach."

What have other doctors learned about hydrochloric
acid therapy? In a three-year collection of articles taken
from *The Medical World,* and written by various physicians, is some sobering information, together with complete case histories. The collection is called *Three Years
of HCL Therapy.** Much of it agrees with Dr. Tuckey's
findings. There is additional and often startling information.

Here are some examples:

Professor A. E. Austin, author of the *Manual of Clinical
Chemistry,* lists these results which can occur in deficiency
or absence of HCL:

1. Gradual and increasing starvation of the mineral
elements.

2. Incomplete digestion and assimilation of food.

3. A septic process of tissues will appear, such as
pyorrhea, dyspepsia, nephritis (kidney disease), appendici-
tis, boils, abscesses, and pneumonia.

4. Stagnation of pancreas and gall bladder, causing
diabetes and gallstones.

Professor Austin thus found the absence or great deficiency of HCL paves the way for all forms of degenerative diseases.

---

* Published by Lee Foundation for Nutritional Research,
Milwaukee, Wisconsin 53201.

Here are statements by other physicians from *Three Years of HCL Therapy*.

Walter B. Guy, M.D.: "Deficiency of this hydrochloric peptic solution must, of necessity, bring about a slow starvation of the mineral elements and imbalance, also a fixation of deposits in various tissues. For instance, as already mentioned, deposits of iron in anemia; deposits of urea and sodium in gout and arthritis; an overplus of sodium in edema; a probable deficiency of potassium in tumor and epitheliomata; also a deficiency of calcium in parathyroidism and some forms of asthma; a lack of chloric acid must be manifest in alkalosis of cancer, tuberculosis and septic infections."

Henry Pleasants, Jr., M.D.: "HCL is a powerful bactericidal agent. Cultures of staphylococci and streptococci and other organisms were destroyed within a few minutes when mixed with a dilution of 1-1000." This led to local application in pistular skin affections. "The effect was so spectacular that its importance is no longer questioned."

Desiderius de Beszedits, M.D., former president of the Federal Sanitary Brigade, Oaxaca, Mexico: "I have used HCL solution injected with never failing results in snake bites. No matter how poisonous the snake may be, the injection and cotton soaked in pure HCL and placed on the site of the bite will control the situation."

L. G. Rowntree, M.D.: "A deficiency of HCL is frequently associated with mental fatigue, persistent worry and strain, especially in persons with unstable psyche. The symptoms are very vague: lack of appetite, fullness after eating, gaseous eructations, and diarrhea is more common than constipation. Pain is absent.

"Moreover, HCL forms with the duodenal membrane a hormone named secretin, which stimulates the pancreas (to form insulin), also formation of bile and activity of gall bladder . . . which reduces sugar in the blood. . . . We can visualize still further a toxic liver, hypertension in the arteries . . . flabby muscles, little strength, boils, abscesses, pus formation. Deficiency of calcium, which means an excess of sodium, and deficiency of potassium essential to the heart beat, all are results of deficiency of HCL."

COMMON QUESTIONS ABOUT HYDROCHLORIC ACID

What Causes a Lack of HCL?

A lack of B vitamins in the diet contributes to the condition. Those found associated with a lack of HCL are B-1 (thiamin), B-2 (riboflavin), B-6, pyridoxine, niacin, choline and folic acid.

Most doctors have long agreed that as people age they manufacture less and less hydrochloric acid. Dr. Tuckey says, "This is one of the reasons why our older people are suffering from anemia. We find, with aging, the tendencies toward arthritis, as well as a slowing down of the liver-pancreatic function. However, this also occurs in some people of earlier ages who can be affected by the emotions of everyday living—you don't like your job, the people next door are not compatible, and so on. We have found in the patients we have treated over the years that the cause was due to a *combination of diet and emotional conditions.*"

Doctors writing in *Three Years of HCL Therapy* are in agreement that emotions and stress are an important factor in producing a shortage of HCL. Walter B. Guy, M.D., said, "Deficiency of hydrochloric acid in the gastric juice under the stress and strain of modern civilization is becoming very common."

Americans are eating faster all the time. A research organization, delving into the restaurant field, has come up with the figures. The majority of American restaurants cater to customers in a hurry.

Professor Austin added as early as 1935, "HCL secretion may be completely suppressed by emotion or worry. In these days of emotional stress or worry, loss of homes, business, income and money we may well fear that in the near future a great increase of degenerative diseases, such as cancer, nephritis (kidney), cardiac and nervous and mental affections most assuredly will occur." His prophecy is proving correct.

Physicians have usually assumed that as people age their manufacture of hydrochloric acid automatically slows down, sometimes ceasing altogether. But today there is evidence that, due to stress, people of all ages are suffering from this affliction. One professional therapist reported that when several babies who were less than robust were given a few drops of HCL, added to their formula, their health improved remarkably.

HOW CAN YOU TELL IF YOU HAVE
AN HCL LACK OR SHORTAGE?

There is, of course, one medical test for HCL measurement. It is not pleasant! It involves swallowing a tube and having your stomach pumped out for an analysis. Personally, I would rather use the trial-and-error method. A more recent test involves the use of dye tablets available through laboratories to doctors. The color of the dye changed by the urine indicates the degree of HCL deficiency.

Dr. Tuckey supplies some further guidelines. After warning that this problem is not a condition to play with, he says, "There are a number of simple ways that you can tell if you do not have enough hydrochloric acid.

"One of the simple symptoms is reported by patients who say, 'Oh, I can't drink fruit juice; it sours my stomach!' This is generally a quick indication of a deficiency of HCL.

"Another symptom is gas and bloating about an hour or two after eating. As I have already said, halitosis is another."

Surprisingly, a loss of taste for meat has been found to be another symptom. Alexander Slanger, M.D., professor emeritus and consultant, New York Polyclinic Medical School-Hospital, in *Geriatrics* (August, 1966) sums up most of the symptoms. He says, "The symptoms of too little HCL mimic the symptoms of too much. They include epigastric pain, distress, fullness, distension, nausea, gas, and diarrhea, vomiting, even severe heartburn.

"The condition now occurs in the younger age and increases with aging."

BEWARE OF ANTACIDS

The lack of hydrochloric acid, masquerading as "too much acid," has apparently become a national malady. The average person, accustomed to stress and tension, a poor diet, hurried eating, and motivated by commercials, carries a supply of antacid tablets handy, believing he has the right remedy.

Adelle Davis writes, "I once heard a doctor lecturing on

nutrition, state that the hydrochloric acid of the stomach was so valuable that every antacid preparation should be prohibited by law."*

She adds, "One physician, reporting in a medical journal, told of a person who had been miserably ill and depressed for 17 years. She had consulted doctor after doctor, all of whom had recognized that she suffered from multiple deficiencies of B vitamins, and one after another had given her individual B vitamins, B complex preparations, liver and liver extracts. Nothing had helped her. When she was finally given hydrochloric acid with each meal, she made a 'rapid and dramatic recovery' in a single week and remained well afterward."

HOW MUCH HCL SHOULD BE TAKEN?

Dr. Tuckey says, "Experimenting with yourself is not the best way to establish whether you have a deficiency of HCL, or what the proper dosage should be. However, I believe the general public is often cut off from the source of information they should have in their everyday life. If you have gastro-intestinal problems, and don't digest your food properly, you should discuss it with your doctor. If you are not satisfied, go to someone who understands the problem. It is something that you should have a complete understanding about, yourself. I have never had a patient in my office during the years I practiced, with whom I did not sit down and explain what his condition was. I would give him the tools to build his house. I wouldn't build it for him, but I would give him the tools and show him how to use them.

"Every once in a while a patient would come into our office with a border-line stomach ulcer because someone had given him hydrochloric acid when he didn't need it. It was an exception, but it happened because some of the symptoms between too much and too little HCL are identical.

"If you already have too much HCL, or if you get too much in your stomach after taking the tablets, drink two or three glasses of water to dilute the excess and the discomfort. *If* the discomfort is a result of taking the tablets, cut your dose in half. If you have a *lack* of hydro-

* Adelle Davis, *Let's Get Well* (New York: Harcourt, Brace and World, 1965).

chloric acid in the stomach and have already experienced a burning, it will disappear when you take the tablets.

"I generally give my patients one hydrochloric acid betaine with pepsin tablet at breakfast and lunch and two with dinner. I do not find apple cider vinegar or lemon juice as effective."

IS HCL SAFE?

Apparently most physicians accept hydrochloric acid as a routine digestant but are unaware of its tremendous potential in treating or preventing various diseases. Judging by the medical literature, very few doctors have conducted serious research on the subject.

Is it safe to take hydrochloric acid? Dr. Tuckey has already given his opinion. Here are other answers from physicians who have thoroughly studied the effects of HCL and reported them in *Three Years of HCL Therapy*.

Burr Ferguson, M.D.: "There is no danger of toxicity since HCL is one of the very few inorganic acids which are normal constituents of the human body."

Walter B. Guy, M.D.: "The remedy can in no wise cause injury. It has curative properties in diabetes, tuberculosis and other degenerative diseases. It will restore the normal acidity of the stomach and this brings about those conditions whereby the digestive organs will absorb the minerals for sustained health."

Dr. Paul Roth, of Battle Creek Sanitarium, adds that he does not use HCL as a medicine, but to replace a lack in the body. He states, "It cures no ailment known to me but simply stimulates all the known and unknown forces of resistance, the same forces that have earned for nature the reputation of being the best of doctors; the same forces which Hippocrates called, 'a vital spirit in all of us, for the corrections of ailments of our kind.'"

DO YOU HAVE TO TAKE HCL THE REST OF YOUR LIFE?

Dr. Tuckey states, "In our early days of working with hydrochloric acid we kept the patients on the tablets indefinitely. We had no other approach to normalizing the HCL in the stomach. But as time passed, particularly in the last five years, we did a lot of testing and we learned that by giving the patient a pancreatic tablet containing duodenal substance together with the hydrochloric acid, we could generally normalize the HCL so that we could take the patient completely off of it in from two to four months."

DOES HCL HELP APPEARANCE?

Definitely, for those who need it! People who are deficient in HCL age quickly, look pale, wan, haggard, and exhausted. Conversely, as they begin to take HCL to correct their deficiency, their drawn and haggard appearance is gradually replaced with a fresh, alert, more youthful expression.

Dr. Tuckey also found that skin rashes and diseases which did not respond to other treatment completely cleared up as a result of HCL therapy.

But more than that, when HCL is coupled with a specific nutrient, it can become a royal road to health and beauty, as you will discover in the next chapter. Hydrochloric acid may well prove to be an undiscovered genie.

The next step in making yourself over is to choose the right repair materials.

7 The Royal Road to Health and Beauty

There is abundant evidence that protein is one of the most important elements necessary for good health and good looks. I am prepared to offer proof to those people who will vigorously challenge this statement. The disturbances which have long been blamed on "too much protein" may turn out to be due to another cause.

I have many vegetarian friends whom I love dearly. They are always trying to convert me. I am unmoved. In reams of research I have found many ill effects on health, and especially on appearance, of too little protein. Furthermore, those who substitute processed carbohydrates (cakes, cookies, candies, and white-flour products) for protein are slowly committing suicide. The reason: carbohydrates build weak cells; protein builds strong, healthy cells.

The U.S. Department of Agriculture Yearbook (1939 edition) states, "If there were one secret of life, protein might be considered at the heart of it, since protein is the essential stuff of which all living tissue is made."

Dr. Vulmiri Ramalingaswami, of the All-India Institute of Medical Science, states that protein deficiency affects the entire body. Different organs are adversely affected at different times. In those organs which have a high rate of cell turnover, such as the liver, pancreas, and salivary glands, the adverse changes take place within a few days. Bone thickness is reduced within fifteen days. Muscles, in which 45 per cent of the body's protein is stored, do not begin to atrophy until much later. Production of new cells slows down sharply. However, when protein is restored, manufacture of new cells resumes and many damaged organs can be repaired, Dr. Ramalingaswami says.

Vegetarianism seems to make people feel better at first. Trouble becomes noticeable usually only after a prolonged deficiency.

One nutritionist who serves on the staff of a medical clinic told me, "I have seen results of a vegetarian diet followed too long by the patients who come to our clinic. The activity of their adrenal glands is subnormal, and there is nerve damage and anemia in nearly every case."

I recently observed a man in his mid-thirties who began to complain of a tingling in his hands and fingers, feet and toes, which soon became unbearably painful. Since his vocation required that he spend many hours a day typing, his work came almost to a halt. A nutritional physician whom he consulted asked him when he first noticed the appearance of the symptoms. The man thought for a moment then answered, "After living on a vegetarian diet for twelve years."

Protein cannot be stored in the body for long. When the supply is depleted the body is forced to feed on itself. George K. Anderson, M.D., of the Council on Foods and Nutrition of the American Medical Association, stated as early as 1954 that the knowledge that protein is a preventive and curative food substance has developed only within the last few years. He added that there are no noticeable effects from a deficient intake of food proteins over a short period of time. Prolonged protein deficiency, however, can cause the following disturbances:

> Anemia
> Kidney disease
> Liver disease
> Peptic ulcer
> Poor wound healing
> Lack of resistance to infection
> Irritability
> Fatigue
> Low blood pressure
> Weakness
> Wasting
> High cholesterol
> Poor circulation
> Constipation
> Mental retardation in children
> Edema (water storage)
> Poor vision

Dr. J. J. Stern of the State Hospital in Utica, New York, says that amino acids (the factors which make up proteins) are essential for the health of an eye lens. He found that a high proportion of laboratory animals, deficient in protein, invariably developed cataracts. If the amino acids were fed to the animals before the condition progressed too far, the cataracts disappeared. In fact, all parts of the body are dependent on it in some way for survival. Melchior T. Dikkers, Ph.D., says, "You must keep this in mind: without protein, life could not go on. No living being survives without protein. The word 'protein,' coined by a Dutch chemist in 1839, means 'of first importance.' The stuff of life. The No. 1 in your life. No protein—no life! Here are some examples:

"To function properly the liver needs protein. It must also receive all the amino acids at one time.

"The hormone, that chemical regulator, is a protein.

"The genes, the controllers of heredity, are proteins.

"The secretion of the thyroid gland is a protein.

"Insulin, produced by the pancreas, is a protein.

"Secretions of the pituitary gland, the master gland of the body, are proteins.

"Antibodies, which defend the body against infection, are proteins.

"All enzymes, which control a multitude of body functions, are proteins.

"Hemoglobin, the red coloring matter of the blood, is a protein.

"If you have a wound, a cut, or a burn, protein is lost in the fluid which escapes. The remaking of healthy tissue over an injury of the body must have protein to repair the damage."

Your muscles, including your heart, liver, kidneys, especially your heart, and even your eyes, are made of protein. Lack of protein weakens muscle tone and makes them flabby. Without it, even your facial muscles will begin to droop and your skin will shrivel and wither. Wrinkles and premature aging appear. Dr. Charles S. Davidson, of Harvard Medical School and Boston City Hospital, has reported that eating more protein may be the way to stop the withering which develops as people grow older.

Adelle Davis describes it this way, "Since your body structure is largely protein, an under supply can bring about age with depressing speed. . . . muscles lose tone, wrinkles appear, aging creeps in; and you, my dear, are going to pot."*

After reading these many needs for protein, please stop to consider: How in the world can your wonderful body machinery operate at peak efficiency without it?

WHY VEGETARIANS HAVE TROUBLE WITH ANIMAL PROTEIN

In 1915, Dr. W. J. Mayo wrote, "If flesh foods are not fully broken up, decomposition results, and active poisons are thrown into an organ not intended for their reception."

One law in nature is that we lose what we do not use. Many investigators have noted that protein-eating stimulates the production of hydrochloric acid. On the other hand, a lack of protein may cause a depletion of HCL. Furthermore, one of the symptoms of a lack of HCL is often a corresponding lack of interest in, or loss of taste for, meat or other animal proteins. Perhaps this is the wisdom of the body trying to tell the person, "Don't eat

* Adelle Davis, *Let's Eat Right to Keep Fit* (New York: Harcourt, Brace and World, 1954).

meat; you can't digest it anyway." Adding HCL to the diet usually solves the problem.

A vegetarian recently sent me pictures of a man taken before-and-after giving up meat eating. The caption under the two pictures stated: "See how much better the man looks who has changed over to a complete fruit diet."

Another vegetarian wrote me telling how much time he had spent in a Veterans' Hospital. He said all manner of things were wrong with him. The medical diagnosis was that his troubles had all come from eating meat. When he was put on a diet of fruits and vegetables, his symptoms began to disappear.

Vegetarians would proclaim with glee, "We told you so. This is proof of the dangers of meat eating!" But they have overlooked another explanation, far more important.

Dr. Tuckey, whom I introduced in the last chapter, asks, "What can you expect, when you have an intestinal sewer stopped up? If you are interested in living, then I say to you: if there is a deficiency of hydrochloric acid and I don't care whether you are a meat eater or a vegetarian, it makes little difference; when there is a deficiency of hydrochloric acid in the stomach, you are not going to break down your food properly or assimilate it properly."

Obviously, toxins from undigested food are going to cause putrefaction. The reason why many people become vegetarians is because they believe that meat does not agree with them, or they "don't feel well" after eating it. But these reactions apparently are not due to the meat but to lack of proper digestion of that meat.

A mother called me recently to tell me about her small son who was suffering from a severe case of diarrhea. She said, "Our pediatrician, a wise elderly woman, told me I must get some acid into him immediately."

The diarrhea had washed away all of his hydrochloric acid and the doctor feared the child might pick up another bacterial infection. To protect him from the possibility the physician gave him a prescription for HCL to compensate for the loss until his own supply built up again.

Thus the toxins, bacteria, and other digestive problems attributed to animal proteins may be actually due to a lack of hydrochloric acid. In condemning meat or any kind of protein we have been probably barking up the wrong tree.

Dion Fortune, the English author, states, "Vegetarianism

has to be thoroughly understood and exceedingly well used if it is to be successful, and even so, there is a goodly proportion of people incapable of digesting vegetable proteins, which are not nearly so easily dealt with as animal substances. Nothing but experience and experimentation can show whether a vegetarian diet suits a given person. Indigestion is not the only indication that all is not well. Loss of appetite, loss of energy, loss of weight, or a flabby stoutness are all danger signals which if disregarded will cause chronic ill-health.

"Vegetarianism may agree with a person well enough at first, but after a considerable period, possibly years, she may find that she is becoming subject to neuritis, neuralgia, sciatica, or one of the nerve pains. This is a sure indication that a vegetarian diet is affording insufficient nourishment, not because it may not contain the necessary food units, but because the digestion is unable to assimilate them and they are passing out of the body unchanged."

A professional woman of my acquaintance bears testimony to the above statement. After being a vegetarian for years she eventually acquired a heart condition which led to several attacks, nearly fatal. She also contracted a serious kidney disturbance. Later she began to suffer from great fatigue. As late as her early seventies she was encouraged to return to a high protein diet, including animal protein, in addition to her usual vegetables and fruits. This change, aided by natural food supplements in liberal amounts to help restore elements missing from her body for so many years, brought about a surprising reformation. Her heart and kidney conditions are now under control, her fatigue has vanished, and her radiant, youthful-looking appearance belies her years.

WHAT KIND OF PROTEIN IS BEST?

Nutritionists consider animal protein superior because it is more similar to human protein. Animal protein also contains all of the 20 amino acids, whereas some plant proteins lack some of the essential amino acids, making it impossible for the body to synthesize protein. Or, if the plant proteins do contain all of the amino acids, sometimes the level of the various amino acids is low. For example, W. Duane Brown, Ph.D., a researcher on protein, agrees that animal proteins are of better quality than vegetable proteins. He finds that cereal proteins are often low in lysine, and in some cases methionine and tryptophane (all amino acids), whereas oil seeds and nuts are often deficient in lysine and methionine. He reports that for man the most important changes found in malnutrition are those due to insufficient intake of protein, or using a protein of poor quality. Animal protein contains vitamin B-12, rarely found in vegetable protein. One study has ascertained that the amount of B-12 in blood serum of vegetarians is lower than in nonvegetarians.

Some plant proteins are preferable to others. The U.S. Department of Agriculture rates the protein content of sunflower seeds almost as high as steak, and higher than all other vegetable seeds. Its protein is 98 per cent digestible, with a utilization value of 64.5 per cent, which places the seeds in the same classification as egg protein. Sunflower seeds can also be used as a reducing food. Sesame seed in meal form is considered as good a protein as soybean meal, although there are differences. Sesame meal is richer in methionine (an amino acid) than any other plant source. It is weak in lysine (another amino acid) where soybean meal is strong. Used together they supplement each other.

Tables showing a protein analysis of nuts are almost nonexistent. Cashews are thought to be a complete protein and the protein of almonds compares favorably with that of meat. All nuts are more nutritious if they are eaten raw.

The best sources of vegetable proteins are légumes (certain peas and beans), seeds, some grasses, and some nuts. The soybean is the most complete protein of all vegetables. Brewers yeast is an excellent high-quality nonmeat protein. But getting enough protein through these sources is often questionable. The late Dr. E. E. Pfeiffer, one of the most outstanding nutrition researchers of our time, explains why all of the essential amino acids, usually found only in animal protein, are so important.

He said, "The absorption of these amino acids is a dynamic process requiring a specific balance. . . . Without them all, the body cannot maintain its balance. Animal feeding experiments have shown that one meal deficient in one or more of the important amino acids cannot be made up for by another meal, even four hours later! For proper utilization, the body needs a complete amino acid balance in each meal. Exactly how to bring this about other than eating animal protein needs quite a knowledge of the biochemistry of food."

For example, gelatin is an incomplete protein and should always be used with a complete protein.

Dr. Pfeiffer added, "For the layman, it is almost impossible to judge the proper amino acid balance. The best and most reliable approach is to eat as many different foods as possible and not to become one-sided in one's eating habits."

The only vegetarian I have ever known who remained healthy, vital, and energetic occasionally ate some fish and fowl and relied heavily on brewers yeast for his protein supply. However, he took a pencil and paper each day and computed his grams of protein intake. If his supply was short, he made up the deficit before going to bed. So now, at bedtime, instead of counting sheep to get to sleep, I count my grams of protein intake for the day, too.

To give you some idea of the amount of protein contained in complete proteins, here is a chart to help you:*

Sources of Complete Proteins	Amounts	Grams of Protein
Soybean flour, low fat	1 cup	60
Cottonseed flour	1 cup	60
Wheat germ	½ cup	24
Brewers yeast, powdered	½ cup	50
Egg	1	6
Milk, whole or skim, buttermilk	1 qt.	32 to 35
Cottage cheese	½ cup	20
American or Swiss cheese	2 slices	10 to 12
Soybeans, cooked	½ cup	20
Meat, fish, fowl	¼ lb. (approx. 1 serving)	15 to 22

HOW MUCH PROTEIN DO YOU NEED?

The amount of protein usually recommended is 1 gram of protein for every 2.2 lbs. of body weight. The Food and Nutrition Board of the U.S. National Research Council recommends 65 grams of protein daily for men; 55 for women (except 65 during pregnancy and 75 during lactation). However, the recommendations of this board for all nutrients are considered low. Adelle Davis believes

* From Adelle Davis, *Let's Eat Right to Keep Fit* (New York: Harcourt, Brace and World, 1954).

that if you have been short of protein for an extended time you need 150 grams daily for at least two months. The findings in other countries call for a higher amount of protein than that recommended in America.

The more energy expended, the more protein is needed. In Sweden, laborers doing hard work were found to need 189 grams daily; Russian laborers, 132; German soldiers, 145; laborers in Italy, 115; in France, 135; and in England, 151. The British Medical Association has decided that the most realistic allowance should be between 80 and 100 grams daily for the average person.

CAN YOU GET TOO MUCH PROTEIN?

If the right type of protein is taken, together with hydrochloric acid, if necessary, normal people do not seem to experience difficulties, even an increase of uric acid, so long considered the bugaboo of meat eating. W. A. Krehl, M.D., Ph.D., of Marquette University School of Medicine, who upholds the use of protein as a means of improving health as well as appearance, explains, "It has long been shown that long exposure to experimental diets low in protein results in extensive skin changes. These changes are characterized by dryness, scaliness, inelasticity, and a gray, pallid appearance, suggestive of old age."

Dr. Krehl is concerned about the growing protein shortage throughout the world. He adds, "The important question here is how to get into the basic diets of millions of people enough protein, particularly of animal origin, of proper nutritional value. This is undoubtedly the single most challenging problem to our nutritionists, economists, agriculturists and public health workers."

Dr. Krehl also believes that edema (a great accumulation of fluids in the body) is associated with protein deficiency, and is usually reversed by adequate amounts of a good dietary protein.

His only warning against too much protein is: "However, in severe cirrhosis of the liver where the ability to metabolize amino acids (the ability to absorb protein properly) is seriously impaired, protein must be used with great caution to prevent the development of hepatic (liver) coma."

This would indicate that if your health is obviously

below par, a check-up by a physician is indicated before going on this or any other similar program.

W. Duane Brown, Ph.D., the protein researcher, states that high-protein diets are probably not deleterious. He adds, "Ingestion of large amounts of protein usually results in increased excretion [of surplus protein]."

CAN ADEQUATE PROTEIN REPAIR DAMAGE?

Yes. There are many laboratory tests as proof. In one study, reported in the *American Journal of Clinical Nutrition* (August, 1968), fourteen patients were found to be suffering from protein deficiency. Their symptoms included:

Anemia
Loss of muscle tone
Generalized edema (water storage)
Diarrhea in some patients
Weakness

Yet some of these patients had been living on a comparatively high protein diet (51 grams daily), but the bulk of the protein had been derived from plant protein, especially wheat.

When all fourteen patients were put on a diet of 100 grams of protein daily, largely animal protein, their hemoglobin improved significantly; diarrhea subsided; and edema and weakness completely disappeared—all within three months, proving that adequate protein can repair damage.

AN ACCEPTABLE SOURCE OF PROTEIN FOR EVERYONE

Probably the greatest boon for easily ensuring a sufficient intake of protein is the new protein powders. Originally developed to provide protein for underdeveloped countries, the idea has caught on and is being used by an increasing number of people in all walks of life with excellent results. These protein powders are not the synthetic "instant breakfasts" or the so-called reducing powders. Instead, they come from natural sources and are often combinations of various vegetable proteins, or vegetable and animal proteins. Athletes are using them. Radio, screen and television personalities are using them, and for good reason. One man told me after using a protein powder for several weeks, "I now have so much energy, I don't know what to do with it!"

Different protein powders seem to serve different purposes. One, which combines brewers yeast, sunflower seeds, fenugreek-seed meal and dulse (a sea plant to supply minerals), is apparently slowing down falling of hair and encouraging regrowth of hair in many cases. Another, a glandular protein powder, is being enthusiastically adopted by more and more people to provide both quick and long-lasting energy. This powder is made of the liver, heart, kidney, brain, stomach, and spleen of carefully selected beef. The success stories resulting from its use are abundant. One woman (whom I know personally) was a wheelchair invalid. Due to this glandular protein powder which she takes several times a day, she now owns a health-food store and is on her feet ten hours a day. She has two hundred other people on it, too.

This woman also experienced a normalizing of high cholesterol, high blood pressure, improvement of all body functions including the thyroid. Her skin became firmer; her hair stopped falling and became shiny and manageable; and splitting nails became hard and long. She says she takes 4 heaping tablespoons every single day, or 60 tablets daily when she travels.

A man who began using this glandular protein powder was overweight (230 lbs.); had high blood pressure (it varied from 190–210); a high cholesterol (400) and suffered from gout. He was refused insurance.

After a period of using the glandular protein his medical check-up found his cholesterol normal and his blood pressure that of a "teenager" (according to the doctor): it was 135 over 80. He is now eligible for unlimited insurance. He has not had a gout attack in years; his energy is tremendous; his nerves, physical and emotional stamina are normal in every way.

Other good results reported by people who have used this glandular protein powder regularly for weeks, months, even years, include a change from extremely wrinkled skin, lifeless hair and flabby flesh, to a wrinkle-free face, healthy hair, and firm, taut body tissue. Anemia and allergies are overcome; blood pressure is lowered to normal, nerves are steadied, and there is usually a dramatic rise in energy level.

A plastic surgeon recommends 10 tablets of this same product plus an animal protein for each of the three meals daily to maintain firm and youthful facial muscles in his clients.

Another protein powder is made of dried milk and eggs, and is combined with fresh milk and raw eggs into an eggnog seasoned with assorted flavorings. Whipping cream is added. Many athletes and winners of "Mr. America" and "Mr. Universe" titles swear by this type of protein.

I can immediately hear cries of protest: "It would make me fat"; "Dairy products are supposed to raise your cholesterol"; "I am allergic to milk—it is mucus-forming"; "I can't eat eggs—my doctor won't let me because they are so high in cholesterol."

Let's handle these protests one by one.

WHY EGGS?

The reason that eggs are used as a source of protein is because they are considered a nearly perfect food. George Briggs, chairman of the nutrition department of the University of California, Berkeley, says the egg is "one of nature's most nearly perfect foods."

The *American Journal of Clinical Nutrition* (May, 1968) adds, "Egg protein is well digested and well utilized." Dr. D. M. Hegsted, a professor of nutrition, Harvard School of Public Health, states, "Egg is the naturally occurring food with the highest biological value (0.94), so that egg is often called the 'ideal food.' Egg also has a high degree of digestibility, i.e. it is completely absorbed in the gastrointestinal tract." (Fertile eggs available from farmers or health stores are considered nutritionally superior.)

WHAT ABOUT MILK?

There is much controversy in health circles over the use of milk. Some nutritionists, including Adelle Davis, recommend it highly, considering it a superior source of protein and calcium. She says, "I have yet to find any person young or old, who can maintain an adequate diet without drinking milk." Others do not agree. Those nutritionists, however, who are in favor of milk prefer raw certified milk and cream to pasteurized.

Adelle Davis admits that many people are allergic to milk and she suggests alternatives: yogurt, acidophilus milk, buttermilk, or goat's milk, which usually do not cause distress. However she warns against soy milk. She says,

"Most physicians agree that soy milk lacks much of the value of cow's milk and should be used as a last resort." Her reasons are that soy milk is seriously deficient in vitamins B-1, B-2, calcium, iodine, and two important amino acids (protein factors), methionine and cystine. She says that these deficiencies can be overcome by the following formula: To 1 quart of water, add 1 cup of full-fat soy flour or powder to which 1/3 *cup of calcium lactate per pound* has been added.

As an example of what milk has done for appearance, *Science News Letter* (April 6, 1968) reported, "Before-and-after photographs of babies transformed from starving creatures into plump laughing youngsters demonstrate the effect of well-balanced protein feeding" from animal protein such as milk.

NO PROVEN CHOLESTEROL HAZARD

Since dairy products contain cholesterol, many people assume that they will elevate cholesterol in the body. Broda O. Barnes, Ph.D., M.D., of Colorado State University, believes that foods high in cholesterol do not cause cholesterol to rise, but that high cholesterol stems from different causes. Many other studies agree. Dr. Barnes believes that the chief culprit in a high cholesterol level is high carbohydrate foods, such as sugar, bread, pastries, which stimulate the liver to produce more cholesterol. He has placed many of his patients on a diet of whipping cream plus raw eggs. Weight and cholesterol both dropped.

Actually the body needs cholesterol for the manufacture of sex hormones, bile, and vitamin D. Even when we avoid cholesterol foods, the liver manufactures it anyway. So those who are mistakenly avoiding eggs and unsaturated oils in order to avoid an increased cholesterol level are apparently headed in the wrong direction. One nine-year study found that people who ate no fat had the highest blood-level fats, whereas those who ate 70 per cent fat had the lowest. Another study showed that when patients ate twelve eggs at a time, fried in unsaturated vegetable oil, their cholesterol showed little or no increase at all!

In still another study conducted by Harvard School of Public Health, and the Loma Linda College of Medical Evangelists, School of Medicine, California, several groups were tested for cholesterol levels. Those who were non-vegetarians (30 per cent of their protein came from meat) had higher cholesterol levels (an average of 291). Lacto-ovo vegetarians (those who eat dairy products but no meat) had a medium level (an average of 256), both readings within the accepted normal range.

HOW TO CHOOSE THE RIGHT PROTEIN POWDER

There are now at least fifty brands of protein powders available in health stores. Read the labels carefully before buying, and then buy the smallest quantity possible before accepting it as a permanent addition to your diet.

There is one caution to observe in using brewers yeast or animal proteins. These foods are high in phosphorus. Calcium, closely associated with phosphorus, needs to be increased for calm and steady nerves or else "phosphorus jitters" may result. This problem is easily corrected. Merely step up your calcium intake when you step up animal protein or protein powders or brewers yeast. Adelle Davis suggests adding to each pound of brewers yeast ¼ cup of calcium lactate powder or ½ cup of calcium gluconate, mixing all well before using. Those people who believe brewers yeast causes gas usually experience relief on taking hydrochloric acid. Brewers yeast can be added to other protein powders, too. I am currently taking equal parts of a glandular protein powder and brewers yeast-plus-calcium.

Protein powders are taken by stirring a heaping tablespoon into juices such as pineapple juice, plain water flavored with black cherry concentrate (available at health stores), or tomato juice. They may be used as between-meal snacks or instead of a meal.

Protein, as you will see in later chapters, plays a role in beauty. The reason: hair, skin, and nails are 98 per cent protein. Thus, if you are protein-deficient your skin and hair and nails will announce the fact. Another symptom of protein deficiency is identified by a washed-out, expressionless look in the eyes and face. It is common in our hippies today.

I learned this lesson the hard way. I "guinea pigged" a milk-and-egg powder, to be used with milk, cream, and an occasional raw egg, because it was producing such wonderful results for many people. To my great disappointment I found that I was allergic to milk, cream, and raw fertile eggs (even though I raise my own chickens). I was forced to substitute another type of protein powder.

If you experience any unusual allergy symptoms, you

may also need to try another protein powder. A rash is not the only allergic symptom. Headaches, irritability, fatigue, even edema may occur. There is a simple do-it-yourself method of discovering your allergies. It is explained by Arthur F. Coca, M.D., in his book* and is completely explained in the allergy chapter in one of my books.** Remember that allergies do not necessarily condemn a product; what works for one person may not work for another.

Don't sell brewers yeast short as a protein powder! With its full array of 10 B vitamins, 18 minerals, and all the essential amino acids, it is a bell-ringer. Morton S. Biskind, M.D., found that when it was coupled with the use of desiccated liver tablets, the combination produced excellent results.***

Protein, therefore, is a must for body health. Even more exciting is the cosmetic effect of protein on skin and hair. Used externally, it can actually help rebuild your skin and your hair, as you will see in a later chapter.

8 Vitamins Are Spark Plugs

We were not meant to be ill or ugly due to poor health. The original plan for life—plant, animal or human—was a perfect plan for perfect health. When a living being was first placed on earth, various forms of nourishment were also placed on earth to properly sustain life and health. According to various references in the Bible, a plant or herb for every possible illness was made available in na-

* *The Pulse Test* (New York: Arc Book, paperback).

** *Get Well Naturally* (New York: Devin-Adair Company, 1965; also, Arc Book, paperback, 1968).

*** Linda Clark, *Stay Young Longer* (New York: Pyramid Books, paperback, 1968).

ture. Even today, birds and animals know and use them. There are almost unbelievable examples of how birds and animals cure themselves with certain foods or medicinal plants.* Botanic therapy—the use of naturally grown, sun-dried tonic and cleansing herbs, roots, leaves, and barks—has played an important role in human health, also, since the beginning of time.

Euell Gibbons, an herb investigator and author of several books on the value of herbs, recently decided there must be some logical explanation for herbal cures. He obtained samples of herbs from fields and forests and offered them to a state university testing laboratory to determine what might be responsible for the value of the herbs. Mr. Gibbons was not surprised when the analyses revealed that herbs, time-honored for centuries in promoting health, contained rich sources of vitamins and minerals. Although the names—vitamins and minerals—were newcomers, the ingredients had always been there, as the Bible states, probably from the beginning of life itself.

Since nature has set up a master plan, or laws, for perfect health, we run into trouble when we break these laws. We were meant to eat pure whole food, breathe pure air, and drink pure water. When we tamper with nature, bypass it, or try to outsmart it, we run into trouble.

WHAT CAUSES ILLNESS?

In ages past, a sick or chronically unhealthy person was an exception. Today just the reverse is true. Do you honestly know many people who don't have at least a little something wrong with them? A backache, a constant headache, fatigue, a sinus condition, insomnia, constipation, "nerves" and irritability, cavities, or a host of other complaints?

Stop and think: What could be the cause? There are two possible explanations. One is that many foreign substances are getting into our bodies through food, air, and water. The other explanation is that the repair materials which should be in the average diet are no longer there in sufficient amounts to keep us healthy. Consequently our individual and national health is becoming increasingly worse. The Metropolitan Life Insurance Company admits

---

* See Linda Clark, *Get Well Naturally* (New York: Devin-Adair Company, 1965; Arc Book, paperback, 1968).

the death rate is climbing, and statistics have shown for some time that the disease rate (cancer, heart disease, diabetes, etc.) is reaching an all-time high.

This should not be! More important, it need not be.

Every day millions of cells in your body become worn out, damaged, or destroyed. Every day your body is trying to replace, rebuild, repair these cells in order to maintain your health and prevent illness. But in order to accomplish this gigantic task it must have sufficient and effective repair materials. The only way your body can get these repair materials is from your diet. There is no other way.

We have already seen the vast number of adulterants allowed in our food under the guise of "protection of food." None of these adulterants existed in the time of our ancestors. Health was also far better then than it is now. The food eaten by earlier generations was natural, whole, untampered-with farm-fresh food to which nothing was added, nothing taken away. Not so today. Food is impregnated with at least 2,500 chemicals, some of which have been proved to be disturbing or actually dangerous to health but are allowed anyway. Also, to make many packaged foods last longer on the shelf without spoilage, fragile vitamins and minerals are removed. Some of this food is "enriched," which means that many natural vitamins have been removed; a few synthetic vitamins have been restored. This plan is not what nature intended and it cannot guarantee health.

Alan H. Nittler, M.D., points out that in our ancestors' time greater physical effort was necessary merely to exist. To supply that physical energy, 6,000 calories were needed daily. These calories also provided the amount of vitamin, proteins, and minerals to maintain good health.

Today it is not necessary to expend as much energy in order to live. Appliances, mechanical devices, cars, and other conveniences require only that we push buttons, turn switches, shift levers. We do not need 6,000 calories for reduced physical activity. In fact, we may gain weight if we eat only half as much. 2,500 calories is the average intake now.

But for total health we still need 6,000 calories worth of repair materials. History has proved that the body stayed well on that amount. Furthermore, because of the stresses of our present civilization, we need more, not less, dietary protection, and we are not getting it. The 2,500 calories the average person eats are "empty" calories, meaning that the nutrients are diluted or displaced by "fillers"; and these nutrients are often synthetic or of inferior quality. Thus the amount of repair materials supplied to the average American today is shockingly low. Vested interests which produce such food deny this. Scientific analysis proves them wrong. Health statistics also prove them wrong.

A six-year survey has revealed that malnutrition affects 999 persons out of 1,000 and that only 2 persons in 2,511 have a perfect diet. The government is alarmed because most families, including children and teenagers, even those who have plenty of money, live mostly on the same old things: hamburgers and hot dogs on white buns; potato chips, soft drinks, sandwiches, and desserts. Although the state of poor health does not become apparent at first, eventually it reflects this diet. Witness the draft status. A completely healthy young man is a rarity. Previous standards are being relaxed in order to fill the draft quota. And the health of teenage girls, our future mothers, is similar. Birth defects in their children is one proof. A few scientists have established without a doubt that many birth defects are a direct result of inadequate body-building materials in the diet of the young mother-to-be.

What is the solution? The 2,500 calories we do eat must include foods with concentrated body-building nutrients. In addition, to make up for the deficit of the remaining 3,500 uneaten calories, we must fortify our diet with natural nutritional supplements known as vitamins, minerals, and amino acids, extracted from natural food, which, in addition to protein, also repair and maintain cells properly. This saves us from eating many pounds of bulk which contains them, and thus from gaining unwanted weight, while we build or maintain optimum health.

VITAMINS ARE SPARK PLUGS

Vitamins act as spark plugs for the body machinery. Together with minerals, they help to ignite the use of the body's fuel, especially if it is "high octane fuel" (nutritionally superior food). Thus vitamins can add pep, increase more lasting energy, and produce that good-to-be-alive feeling.

It is only logical that when we eat food which has had the natural vitamins removed we need to restore those vitamins to our diets in supplement form.

This is no longer debatable. More and more people are

discovering the good effects of vitamins. More and more doctors are prescribing them. This explains why thousands of people became enraged when the government's Food & Drug Administration (FDA) decided that Americans should not be allowed to take so many vitamins, particularly in higher-than-average potencies. The potencies they planned to allow were a mere fraction of those which most of us use. According to experts, people who live and work under stress conditions *need* high potency vitamins!

IS THERE DANGER OF TAKING TOO MANY VITAMINS?

Barbara Cartland, nutrition columnist in England who leads many people to better health via the nutrition route, says, "The answer is NO. You can't take too many natural vitamins, which are food, not medicine. They are what should be on your plate, but owing to modern conditions—chemicals in the soil, the air, the water, as well as vitamins destroyed by processing, refrigerating and bad cooking—they are missing.

"You must therefore supplement your diet. You eat every day. You therefore take your vitamins every day. It's not really a lot. Put all you eat in one day in a bucket, and put the vitamins you need in a small saucer. You will then see how few you have taken in proportion to all you consume."

Because so many vitamins are needed in so many parts of the body, I am always shocked when someone proudly announces that he or she is taking just a single vitamin, as if this would solve all their problems, past, present, and future. One vitamin is a very small drop in a very large bucket. Nutritionally speaking, everything is needed to work together for health.

Dr. N. Ethan Edgington, of Harvard, a nutritionally educated physician, considers the fear of taking too many vitamins sheer bubble-headedness. He says, "Can science today say that our hypothetically healthy well-fed child would derive no benefit from a properly balanced vitamin supplement? Emphatically science cannot. . . .

"For my part, I would like to see parents make room in their food budget for vitamin supplements for their children. Any number of foodless foods could well be cut out—candy, pastry, sugar, cornflakes (approximately as nutritious as the box they come in), jelly, crackers, soda pop. [These foods do not contain sufficient, if any, repair materials.]

"But then the best infant supplement I've seen costs about 25¢ a week. Surely a quarter of weekly nutritional insurance is not going to break anyone up in these sunny days."

SURPRISING PROOF OF VITAMINS

Let me tell you a true story about a horse. A friend of mine wanted a safe horse for her two small children to ride. Some neighbors who were moving away were willing to sell their somewhat elderly mare, named "Mother," and my friend bought her.

Several months later the original owners returned to visit Mother and were shocked at her appearance. "She looks awful," they said. "Call the vet, quickly."

My friend, unfamiliar with horses, was surprised. She hadn't noticed anything unusual about Mother's appearance but she did promise to call the vet. Now veterinarians, except for extreme emergencies, improve the health of animals through diet, not drugs. If the animal's coat lacks sheen, or it has little energy, the vet uses the dietary approach to correct the condition. So when my friend phoned the local vet, he asked questions about Mother's appearance and activity.

"Do you give her vitamins?" he asked.

My friend was surprised. "No," she answered. "Am I supposed to?"

"If you want a beautiful, frisky animal, you do," he answered.

So he outlined a diet. It was to include certain amounts of alfalfa (a whole, natural food); oats (another whole, natural, high-protein food); and in case some of the necessary repair material might be missing from these foods, he added a third natural product which included a combination of many grains, proteins, minerals, and vitamins. On top of all that he prescribed, daily, 4 ounces of a vitamin-mineral supplement.

In two weeks you would not have recognized that horse! Her dull coat had become shiny. She held up her once-droopy head. The children exclaimed, "Before, we couldn't get Mother to move fast at all. Now she wants to trot and gallop." The entire family was surprised.

Sometime later they decided to take Mother on a pack

trip. To be sure Mother would have enough energy to
make it, they doubled, on their own, Mother's vitamin-
mineral supplement. And as they did, her energy doubled.
She completed the pack trip with perfect ease.

The family no longer needs to be convinced of the worth
of vitamins. They have witnessed the results in Mother.
They take natural vitamins, too.

What we know about nutrition in people, we have first
learned from animals. People react in the same way.

In the *Health Bulletin* (March 21, 1964), this news item
appeared: "The Chicago Cubs will bolster their baseball
prowess this season with a nutritional drink containing the
B vitamins, niacin, riboflavin, the minerals, iron, and other
nutrients. It's the same milk-shake type supplement that
was approved by the National Aeronautics and Space Administration for use by astronauts on a moon jaunt.

"Bob Whitlow, the Cubs' athletic director, hopes to
convince the boys that they should replace their usual hot
dog and coke snacks with the supplement. 'This stuff gives
the player quick energy with minimum bulk,' he explained."

WHAT VITAMINS ARE HELPFUL?

There is so much scientific proof of health improvement
through the use of vitamins it would now fill not one, but
many books. New information is coming out of scientific
laboratories almost daily. Here is merely a quick digest of
scientific reports to give you an idea of some of the wonderful effects of vitamins. Check the list to see if you have
any of the symptoms.

Vitamin A:

—has helped vision, particularly night blindness which
   causes you to grope haltingly when you go from bright
   light into a dark theater. It also prevents that miserable
   glare reaction from oncoming car lights during night
   driving.
—has produced a feeling of zest for living. It is a real
   perker-upper.
—has added sheen to skin and hair; prevented skin blemishes, even wrinkles due to dryness.
—has helped protect against infections and colds.

It is true that vitamin A is one of the two vitamins
which, taken in excess for some people only, *might* cause

mild disturbances. These cease when the dosage is lowered. Furthermore, if the source of vitamin A is natural, it is apparently safe, regardless of dosage, according to Robert A. Peterman, M.D., writing in the *Journal of the American Medical Association* (December, 1962).

The Vitamin B family (also known as vitamin B complex):

—is one of the backbones of health, energy, well-being, and good looks.
—helps decrease mental confusion.
—is used by the Russians as a natural tranquilizer.
—helps fatigue and insomnia.
—checks irritability. Children given plenty of vitamin B complex are less fussy. Husbands (and wives) who overdrink alcohol are less nervous, irritable, and easier to live with.
—people who take a bountiful supply of vitamin B complex don't have so much trouble "getting going" in the morning.
—the possibilities of the vitamin B complex are almost endless.

Vitamin E: *

—has prevented miscarriages.
—given in proper amounts has got heart patients out of bed and back to mowing lawns.
—has helped childless couples conceive after all else has failed.
—has improved male virility.
—has turned cranky menopausal and premenstrual women into comparative lambs.
—has increased circulation and improved cold feet as well as memory.
—has dramatically helped to remove pain from a sprain.
—has helped to dissolve blood clots naturally and safely.
—by external application, as well as internal use, has healed burns and absorbed scars of many types.
—a deficiency of vitamin E has been found to be involved in many disturbances including liver degeneration, nerve and brain disturbance, anemia, and muscular dystrophy.

Recently I met two friends, a man and a woman, both

---

* See Linda Clark, *Stay Young Longer* and *Get Well Naturally*.

nutritional workers, who looked so much better than when I had seen them six months earlier, I asked for their secret. They told me, "We're taking more vitamin E. We found we weren't taking enough. We have stepped our daily intake up to 800 units."

According to vitamin E experts, large doses do not cause side effects, except possibly in high blood pressure. In this case the experts advise starting slowly and working upward until the correct dose is determined for that person (a nutritional doctor can help you here).

Each person may need a different amount of vitamin E. I know some heart patients who, to control heart pain and shortness of breath, take from 900 to 1,200 units a day. The average dose suggested by the government is only 30 units. It is far cheaper than questionable drugs. It is derived from, but has been removed from, most of our cereals, bread, and flour by refining. This may explain one reason for the shocking rise of heart disease in this country.

Vitamin D:

—helps strengthen the bones of adults as it has helped to control rickets in children.
—used with calcium or vitamin A, both of which are copartners, it has helped some cases of arthritis and bone disease.

Vitamin D is the other vitamin (in addition to vitamin A) which, if taken in excess, for some people might cause temporary disturbances. These disappear when the vitamin is stopped or dosages lowered.

In addition to a very few foods, and in supplement form, vitamin D can also be acquired from exposure to sunshine. It is manufactured in the oil of the skin, but can be washed off with cold water.

When I moved to California I noticed that most of the women were vital and healthy looking, whereas a few, and most men, did not exhibit this healthy vitality. I believe I discovered the reason.

People who spend time outdoors in the summer look healthier than they do in the winter when they are cooped up inside. Most people in colder climates become paler and paler during the winter. This is because even if they are outdoors a lot, in many climates winter sunshine produces no vitamin D. Since vitamin D occurs in so few foods, house-bound as well as office-bound people do not get any vitamin D at all. For instance, student nurses in Michigan working indoors, even in the summertime, were found to have no vitamin D in their blood streams. Yet another study reported that factory workers who ate their lunch outdoors acquired sufficient vitamin D for health on their face, neck, and arms during the lunch hour alone.

Apparently, because of California's year-round summer-type climate, many women spend more time outdoors, whereas other women and men, even in the same climate, are confined to their offices and do not get enough of the sunshine vitamin. One remedy for them is to take vitamin D in supplement form. In proper amounts there is no danger.

Adelle Davis, the well-known nutritionist, says, "The fear of vitamin D toxicity has become so great that I feel there is grave danger in getting too little rather than too much. The 400 units daily recommended by the National Research Council has been shown to be inadequate for adolescent girls; for persons with porous bones; and during illness, when the need for Vitamin D is increased by stress."*

Recent information has been released showing that vitamin D may not be as harmful as claimed. Vitamin D has also been found to help synthesize protein and to incorporate the mineral magnesium into bone structure.

Vitamin C:

Vitamin C is one vitamin I hope never to be without. I have personally experienced, as well as witnessed in many others, near-miracles from its use. One form of vitamin C, ascorbic acid, used in massive amounts can be used as a natural antibiotic, as attested to by several respected physicians.** For example, they found it can stop a beginning cold in its tracks, rout fevers, overcome food poisoning or diarrhea in record time.

One of my friends who travels on research expeditions in out-of-the-way countries finds that as long as he is equipped with handfuls of high-potency ascorbic acid tablets he remains well, while his traveling companions

---

* Adelle Davis, *Let's Get Well* (New York: Harcourt, Brace and World, 1965).
** Linda Clark, *Get Well Naturally.*

contract one ailment after another. Yet the government is trying to stop us from getting these high-potency vitamin C tablets.

An athletic coach says, "I have had some of my boys who were on the verge of a cold take as high as 1,000 milligrams of vitamin C (ascorbic acid) per hour; in some instances 2,000. These measures [taken during the week] would check the cold so that by Saturday they were in competition running the 440, the mile, or the two mile, and running them successfully."

Like the vitamin B group, vitamin C is a family, too. Ascorbic acid is only one member. The complete C family, or complex, is known as the "bioflavonoids." Taking the entire complex on a day-to-day basis has produced these surprising results. It has:

—diminished pain in bursitis in 24 hours and completely eliminated it in 72 hours.
—stopped bleeding of ulcers in 24 to 36 hours.
—prevented miscarriages.
—controlled colds and serious respiratory diseases. The dosage varied from 300 mg. to 1,200 mg. daily of bioflavonoids coupled with vitamin C (ascorbic acid).

A Florida doctor told me that by taking six bioflavonoid capsules (about 350 mg.) daily before the sniffle season begins he is able completely to avoid getting the colds his patients bring to the office.

Again, the government agency, the FDA, is trying to prevent the public's use of these substances derived from natural foods.

Bioflavonoids, used with ascorbic acid (4 to 9 doses a day of 100 mg. of each), were found in a dental study to improve or completely heal 190 out of 200 cases of bleeding gums.

One woman, only twenty-nine years old, had bleeding gums and foul breath. After four weeks of bioflavonoid therapy (9 capsules daily) her gum-bleeding and bad breath disappeared. A postnasal drip also cleared up.

Another patient had tender gums and loose teeth. Bioflavonoids-plus-calcium helped her teeth to tighten remarkably within two weeks.

Those doubters who claim vitamin C does not work probably have not taken enough or for a long enough period of time.

NEW SURPRISES FROM AN OLD VITAMIN

Here are the stories of two other vitamins which should be able to help you or someone in your family. One is new; the other has been with us for some time but has been largely ignored. The latter is vitamin B-6 and it took a general physician from Texas, John M. Ellis, M.D., to unearth and write a fascinating book about some exciting results of using it.*

Dr. Ellis found out, quite by accident, that his patients who complained of tingling and numbness in fingers and toes (particularly while lying down) or who had excruciating cramps in the calves of their legs, were freed from these symptoms within two or three weeks by taking 50 milligrams of B-6 daily. Furthermore, these same patients, without cutting calories, began losing unnecessary weight or inches. Even cattlemen who rode the Texas range on large cattle ranches found they were able to tighten their belts to the last notch without changing their diets. And women, who usually store water during pregnancy, menopause, or the pre-menstrual period, no longer suffered from this problem as long as they continued to take B-6. Many of Dr. Ellis' patients lost up to 3 inches in the waistline within a few short weeks. When B-6 was stopped, the good results ceased.

Dr. Ellis finally learned the reason: B-6 apparently works together with, and sets up a body balance of, two minerals, sodium and potassium, which regulate the body fluids.

Dr. Ellis also learned that vitamin B-6 produced some degree of success in hypertrophic arthritis. Little spurs on the sides of the fingers became painless and finger-swelling disappeared. When the mineral potassium was added to B-6, the combination helped reverse bursitis. This is another example of how vitamins and minerals work together.

After reading Dr. Ellis' book, I became intrigued. What else did vitamin B-6 accomplish? Upon further research, to my astonishment, I found that B-6 has helped relieve burning feet, epilepsy, one form of anemia, male sexual disorders, and is also involved in insomnia, pancreatitis, eczema, loss of hair, slow learning, and some forms of

* John M. Ellis, M.D., *The Doctor Who Looked at Hands* (New York: Vantage Press, 1966).

visual disturbance as well as high cholesterol. Because vitamin B-6 is helpful to the nerves, Dr. Ellis feels it could be used to help prevent heart disorders involving nerves, such as angina.

Vitamin B-6 is also involved in the toxemia of pregnancy, and has been used to alleviate "morning sickness." This little publicized vitamin is also needed to help the body utilize proteins and fats. Without it the body cannot manufacture red blood cells properly and the nervous system is unable to function normally. Dr. David B. Coursin, of St. Joseph's Hospital in Lancaster, Pennsylvania, stated that infants with symptoms of vitamin B-6 deficiency respond to this vitamin dramatically. He reported, "Administration of 100 mg. of vitamin B-6 corrects the biochemical, electrophysical and clinical signs in children within minutes."

This vitamin is naturally present in vegetables and meat but researchers are becoming convinced that a high percentage of people in the U.S. do not get enough B-6 in their diets, and that supplementation may be necessary. This is particularly true, they feel, for those who eat a high protein diet, since B-6 is needed for utilization of amino acids, the building blocks of protein (*Science News Letter*, Nov. 30, 1968).

Vitamin B-6 is destroyed by 245-degree heat. Dr. Ellis, reporting in *Natural Food and Farming* (September, 1967), writes, "Pecans are one of the richest sources of Vitamin B-6 and in a form that is not only edible but appetizing.

"By giving my patients twelve raw pecans daily, I learned that a form of painful neuritis and arthritis of shoulders, arms, and hands could be relieved in six weeks. I have observed patients who ate 12 pecans daily for as long as a year."

Parkinson's disease, another nervous disorder, often called shaking palsy, causes some people's hands to shake. Dr. Douw G. Steyn, of the University of South Africa, says, "To my knowledge, there have, from time to time, been reports in the medical literature on the treatment of this malady with Vitamin B-6 (also known as pyridoxine). One case of Parkinsonism of very long standing (approximately twenty-five years) responded to treatment with this vitamin by injection within two months."

The mineral magnesium also helps to eliminate hand shakiness.

Dr. Miriam Benner reports that massive doses of vitamin B-6 produced incredible improvement in a woman who was paralyzed. The woman had become paralyzed on the left side of her body as the result of an operation. She was given a dose of 2,000 mg. daily of B-6, starting two and one-half years after the operation. According to Dr. Benner, it produced "fantastic, unexpected and rapid improvement" (*Journal of the American Medical Women's Association*, November, 1964).

The many disturbances which vitamin B-6 improves are common in this country. Dr. Ellis explains why: most Americans are deficient in vitamin B-6, he says. The vitamin is largely found in raw or unrefined food. Most of the American diet is cooked or refined and B-6 is processed out of it.

Dr. Ellis' patients showed no side effects of taking 50 mg. of vitamin B-6 daily even after three years.

A NEW VITAMIN

A newly discovered vitamin, B-15, or Pangamic acid, is also accomplishing wonders. The Russians are using it with great success. Coupled with vitamins A and E into a single product, they report that heart pains, shortness of breath, and related weakness have been found to disappear within ten days. Blood pressure has been reduced in some cases, and cholesterol is often dramatically lowered within a short time. Enlarged liver has been reduced to normal. They found that there were no side effects if taken up to 90 mg. daily. Yet this vitamin is being banned in the U.S.!

Since vitamin B-15, though considered non-toxic by true scientists, is not allowed to be sold separately, it can be found in the following foods: brewers yeast, liver, rare steak, edible seeds and sprouted seeds, and brown rice.

The foregoing discussion in this chapter is just a bird's-eye view of some of the values of a few vitamins. You will find more help on what-vitamin-to-use-for-what in my other books, *Stay Young Longer* and *Get Well Naturally*, as well as in other health books.

HOW TO TAKE VITAMINS

There are general rules which should be observed when you take vitamins. Because vitamins are usually highly concentrated, it is wiser not to take them on an empty stomach. Take them with or after meals. Also, don't be deluded into thinking you can get enough of everything you need in a single, small, multiple-vitamin-mineral tablet or capsule. Even though concentrated, there simply is not room for everything you need in one such little droplet. You will find, on reading your labels, that the usual dosage recommended is several a day, and the potencies listed on the label refer to that specific number, not to a single recommended tablet or capsule.

WHAT KIND OF VITAMINS ARE BEST?

Nutrition is a young science. We have only scratched the surface. There are many nutrients and elements which have not yet been identified in the laboratory. And there are so many unknown but necessary interrelationships between nutrients that scientists have not begun to learn them all, let alone apply them to health. John J. Miller, Ph.D., a biochemist who has spent nearly a lifetime studying this subject, believes that man does not know as well as nature all of the elements which exist in plants and natural food, nor how these known and unknown elements are combined in a natural balance of vitamins, minerals, and amino acids (proteins). He says, "We simply do not know enough, nor will we ever be able to improve upon nature's plan of enzyme interrelationships."

Scientists stoutly maintain that synthetic vitamins are exactly the same as natural ones. When a single vitamin substance is known and analyzed it can be duplicated synthetically. However, the unknown elements which accompany these isolated nutrients in natural form may not be present in the synthetic form because many of them have not yet even been discovered or identified. For instance, fish cannot live in synthetic sea water. But when even a small amount of natural sea water is added to synthetic sea water, fish thrive in it. For this reason a natural vitamin, mineral, or food which contains a full supply of known, as well as unknown, substances is a better value, and a richer and more effective source of nutrition.

This does not mean that synthetics are useless. They have their place. Many doctors find that massive doses of a synthetic vitamin or mineral (often by injection) may nudge or stimulate a sluggish cell or laggard organ back into action. But once this is accomplished, continued doses of a synthetic can act as a drug, similar to whipping a tired horse. In the opinion of many nutritionists and nutritionally oriented doctors, once better health has been achieved by a temporary use of synthetics, continued success will be safer, and illness be prevented, by a maintenance use of natural vitamins and minerals derived or condensed from natural foods or plants, and therefore whole, not partial, sources of nutrition.

DO NUTRITIONAL SUPPLEMENTS REALLY WORK?

Do vitamins help people feel better? Do they (plus minerals and protein) help to improve health, even if it has often been seriously affected? More and more people are experiencing the good effects of nutritional supplements. The word "vitamin," practically unknown fifty years ago, is now a household word, and results speak for themselves. Wherever I go, as I lecture throughout the United States, hundreds of people tell me that they have had disturbing health conditions reversed by a good diet plus the use of nutritional supplements. As I explained earlier, I am an example of such health improvement myself. Here is a sample letter from my files which shows the good results achieved through nutrition.

Case 1

One woman, a mother of three small children, wrote:

I have been physically ill and mentally depressed for a long, long time. I was resigned to my condition. Then, quite by accident, I came upon a health food store and one thing led to another.

My life has changed and I am so excited I can't read enough about nutrition or learn enough about health. I stopped drinking coffee, smoking, and eating processed foods. I take the whole alphabet of vitamins from A to Z. I suddenly realized my system was badly depleted in minerals, so I added them, too.

As soon as I started increasing raw foods in my diet and taking over 35 tablets of nutritional supplements daily, my stiffness began to disappear. Now I can get out of the bathtub by myself, which I had not been able to do for two years. I am no longer depressed. My health is becoming better every day.

I get down on my knees and thank God that I discovered health and health products.

Here are case histories from the files of an M.D. who, though trained as an orthodox physician, has shifted over to nutritional therapy (medical language has been purposely included for benefit to other physicians):

Case II

A.T., a 42-year-old male musician, presented himself on June 20, 1952, with an Eczematoid Dermatitis of the right ear, continually present for 12 years, with pronounced nausea for six years, during periods of exacerbation. Uticarial reactions followed penicillin injections. Aureomycin kept dermatitis from severe flare-up.

Prior to June 20, 1952, he had been on daily doses of 3 gr. thyroid for several years. X-ray therapy had been employed elsewhere. Numerous vitamin and mineral preparations had been used. Petrolatum gave relief for years. His diet resembled that of the average American, consisting of dry cereals, homogenized milk, coffee and cream, refined sugar, toast, rolls, occasional fruit juices, sandwiches, soups, and carbonated beverages. Dinners were adequate, and pastries were often the dessert.

Upon recommendation from others, he changed his diet to conform with good nutritional practices. No changes were noted.

Physical examination revealed the following: Chronically inflamed lichenified eczematous right external ear. The face showed superficial erythema extending to the eyelids. All nails and their beds were dystrophic with fissured eczema present on several fingers. This had existed for several years.

Laboratory Reports: Urinalysis: Indican 2+, Sugar 1+, Bacteria 2+, Specific Gravity 1.008, Mucus, and many shreds. Blood analysis: Leucocytes (WBC) 10,600. Differential; Neutrophiles 75 (Stab 1, Segmented 74), Basophiles 2, Eosinophiles 3, Monocytes 2, Lymphocytes 18; Amino Acid Nitrogen 10.4 mg%; Cephalin-Cholesterol-Flocculation 2+, Icterus Index 14.50; Protein-bound Iodine 4.0 mcg%.

He was placed on whole bile, pancreatic, gastric, and intestinal enzymes, Glutamic Acid Hydrochloride, kelp, cold-pressed cod liver oil, crude liver, yeast, dulse, rice bran concentrate, wheat germ oil, and lecithin, as well as papaya in powdered form. Several months were required for complete healing of the ear. Use of petrolatum was continued. No other change in local therapy.

His dandruff, nails, fingers, bowel action and mental status were improved. In addition, he had the ability to add another occupation, Real Estate. He is thriving on the supplements. Laboratory checkup in 3 months was normal, but upon reduction or stoppage of supplements, slight recurrences took place. However, at present time, he is on ⅓ of the original supplementation dosage with no flare-ups.

Case III

L.K., a 39-year-old male, had experienced insomnia for many years, and showed poor resistance. When tired, he would consume alcohol by the pint. Barbiturates caused him to "go out of his mind." Navy discharge papers showed arrested pathological processes in both lung apices, following 2½ months bed rest. He received crude liver, concentrates of Vitamins A, D, B and C complexes, gastrointestinal enzymes, and large quantities of apple juice. These brought him out of his "binges" rapidly.

Here are two other case histories, written by patients themselves, in their own words, but confirmed by two M.D.s for each case.

Case IV

Some eight years ago I was afflicted with arthritis. I had lost most of the use of my right hand and arm. My spine was so affected that it interfered with my ability to get insurance. My knees were also giving me trouble and at times it was difficult to walk.

The doctors were giving me shots in the joints and other treatment. Except for temporary relief from pain the condition did not improve.

About that time a friend of mine told me about a product made from sea plants and vitamins and another made from alfalfa.

A few weeks after I started using the products my joints began freeing up and the pain left. Today there is no sign of any arthritis! I am able to bowl again and I am physically very active.

I feel wonderful and I shall always be grateful for these wonderful natural products.

Case V

I have been anemic since childhood. Due to the anemia it has been necessary for me to have liver and iron shots when my hemoglobin would drop.

As I grew older, the anemia became more severe. About six years ago, at the age of seventy, the anemia was such that I was unable to do much; I was having dizzy spells, my heart was beating fast and I was weak and tired.

The doctors were doing all they could for me to bring up my blood hemoglobin but the condition became worse. I learned about a supplement containing natural vitamins and minerals. Immediately after starting to use it I began to feel better.

Three weeks later I went back to my doctor. He became quite excited discovering that my hemoglobin had climbed from 50 to 90% and I was feeling wonderful!

My dizziness disappeared, my heart doesn't bother me anymore and I never get tired like I used to.

My husband also has had a fine experience with these supplements. He was unable to work because of his heart. After using them he became very much improved. He is now holding down a steady job and he feels fine.

I believe this experience has been an answer to prayer and I thank God for nutritional supplements.

Rheo H. Blair deserves special credit for his over-all concept of nutrition for body improvement. He feels that too many people find one or two "gimmicks" and feel that is enough. Blair uses in his "transformation program," as he calls it, not only a protein powder, but every vitamin supplement known, plus a generous use of calcium, liver extract, and hydrochloric acid. Before-and-after pictures of his subjects show them looking ten years younger, with firm beautiful skin, and normalized weight. He has to his credit many television stars whom you see on your screen every day.

Vitamins are wonderful. But something still more is needed, as the next chapter will prove.

9 Forgotten Magic

Vitamins are not the only route to health. Their appearance is comparatively recent and has eclipsed something far more important: minerals. As one biochemist said, "Whatever a vitamin can do, a mineral can do better. The time is coming when we will realize that minerals are far more important than vitamins."

Charles Northen, M.D., once said, "It is not commonly realized that the vitamins control the body's appropriation of minerals. In the absence of minerals, vitamins have no function. Lacking vitamins, the system can make some use of the minerals, but lacking minerals the vitamins are useless."

John L. Johnson, writing on "Minerals and Health," adds, "To obtain the most benefit from vitamins, *a balanced intake of minerals and amino acids (protein) is imperative.*" He cites many cases where inorganic minerals were fed animals and humans, with either disturbing results, or none at all. When, however, minerals in natural organic forms were used, health flourished.

I will tell you later in this chapter some of the exciting results in the health of many, many people who added minerals to their diet. Scientists first discovered the value of minerals in the health and appearance of plants. Ailing, spindly, and droopy plants have been returned to health again and again by feeding them minerals via the soil (the source of their diet). There are literally thousands of before-and-after pictures to prove this phenomenon. You have probably seen some yourself in gardening books and magazines. Plants properly nourished with minerals are also known to resist disease better than those which are mineral-deficient.

Prior to occupying my present home, I lived on rented property until my own house was ready for occupancy.

On this land was an orange bush. It was puny, sickly, bug-ridden, and what few leaves it still had were diseased and dropping. Needless to say it bore no oranges. I learned from the owner that he had "sprayed and sprayed" to no avail.

A friend came by one afternoon. When she saw the pitiful bush she said, "Oh, I had one in the same condition. I fed it citrus food and in about two months it became luxuriant."

I immediately bought and applied the same type of food. Not only did the bush recover but it began to bear pro-lifically and was able to resist all bugs without spraying. Curious, I read the label on the plant food container and found the mineral content high.

Another friend has a red maple tree which developed a fungus growth. A tree expert diagnosed the trouble as a deficiency of trace minerals (so-called because they occur in minute traces or amounts). When he punched holes in the soil around the tree trunk and fed the tree liberal amounts of trace minerals, it began to recover.

"What about people who lack trace minerals?" I asked this friend. He looked startled. "I never thought of that," he said.

Animals are affected by the lack of minerals, too. In one section of the country, sheep had lustrous coats and were healthy. Less than ten miles away, other sheep were less healthy with poor, scraggly coats. Yet the species of sheep, the climate, and the forage which they ate were the same. Children living in the same area where the healthy sheep grazed were also healthy. In the district where the sheep were ailing, the children were found to be anemic.

The mystery was finally solved when scientists tested the soil and found one-tenth as much iron, one-half as much copper and one-fifth as much phosphorus and cal-cium in the soil as that which produced healthy animals and children. Like the house that Jack built, the soil feeds the plants, which feed the animals (or people). Thus poor soil can produce illness; good soil, health.

You may read in magazines and newspapers that the soil-health relationship is pure myth, and therefore untrue. I disagree.

You need not take my word for it. If you want to take the trouble to write to the U.S. Department of Agricultural Experiment Stations, the soil departments of large universi-ties, and soil scientists, you will find that scientists there have learned from numerous studies that there is a direct connection between the health of the soil and health of plants, animals, and people.

Dr. E. C. Auchter, a former chief of Plant Industry, U.S. Department of Agriculture, explains, "When the plants are consumed by man or animals, the nutrients become part of their bodies. . . . The minerals and other substances absorbed by the plant from the soil, water or atmosphere . . . help to make up such compounds as proteins, fats, vitamins, and other growth regulatory factors.

"In the past, serious bone, skin, digestive and nervous disorders, among other maladies, occurred in certain localities. It is now known that many of these troubles resulted from restricted diets or from eating plant or animal products produced on soils either deficient in certain elements (minerals) or containing elements injurious to health."

Dr. Firman E. Bear, of the Department of Agricultural Chemistry at Rutgers University, made history by proving with an X-ray-type machine on 204 samples of vegetables you and I eat, that depleted soil yielded depleted vegetables, despite the fact that the species, growing season, and harvesting time were identical. What does this mean to you and me? It means that a carrot or a stringbean can look perfectly normal to the naked eye, yet, due to the soil on which it was raised, may be nutritionally impoverished. As Dr. Auchter points out, we humans eat this food, good or bad, build it into our bodies, and improve or suffer accordingly.

Unfortunately you and I do not have X-ray eyes. Nor do we own the type of X-ray machine used by Dr. Bear. When we shop at the supermarket we have no way of knowing what kind of nutrition we are buying and putting into our own and our families' bodies. This is one reason for this book: to help you bypass this problem and show you what to do in order to assure good health.

HOW DO FOOD AND SOIL BECOME DEFICIENT?

Some soil is poor to begin with. Other soils have been overcropped. According to T. M. Rudolph, Ph.D., this is what happens when a farmer grows 100 bushels of corn on an acre of soil. These are the amounts of minerals taken from the earth in order to produce good corn:

125 pounds of potassium
 30 pounds of phosphorus
 50 pounds of magnesium
 20 pounds of sulphur
  2 pounds of iron
3/50 pounds of boron
 ⅓ pound of manganese
Trace of copper
Trace of iodine
Trace of zinc

Dr. Rudolph explains, "Unless the farmer replaces the minerals which he takes from the soil, in the crops which he raises, eventually the soil goes broke. The farmer who continually removes minerals from the soil and never replaces them is not a farmer—he is a miner. Or to put it another way, the soil is like your bank account; you can't keep drawing on it and never make a deposit. Sooner or later the supply runs out and the soil will cease to bear crops."

There is another reason for mineral deficiency in our soil and foods: soil erosion. As the water run-off races to creeks, rivers and eventually the sea, it takes with it precious minerals. Thus the oceans are becoming richer, while the land is becoming poorer. The ocean serves as a mixing bowl of these minerals. Each cubic mile of ocean contains an estimated 200 million tons of minerals! This explains why many land plants and animals have been found mineral-deficient, and no ocean plant or animal has been found deficient! The health of both is excellent.

TRACE MINERALS CAN HELP YOUR HEALTH

Dr. William H. Sebrell, Jr., chairman of the Committee on Recommended Dietary Allowances, National Academy of Science, National Research Council, explains how trace minerals (those which occur in small amounts only) can help your health. He states, "These trace elements are found in minute quantities in the soil, plant, and animal tissues. It is now known that they play essential roles in maintaining cell metabolism and regulating glandular functions. . . . Sometimes individuals fail to get enough of these in their food. . . . In such cases serious illness can result, but just as often or oftener, the result may be lowered efficiency, nervousness or lack of energy. Too vague for any specific diagnosis, such generalized malaise may weaken the individual's capacity throughout much of his lifetime."

And if a lack of trace or minor minerals can cause illness, think what can happen when the major minerals, such as calcium, phosphorus and iron are in short supply. For example, Government Document #264 states: "The soil around a certain Midwest city is poor in calcium. Three hundred children in this community were examined and nearly 90% had bad teeth, 69% showed affections of nose and throat, swollen glands, enlarged or diseased tonsils." More than a third had defective vision, round shoulders, bow legs, and anemia.

A number of years ago Charles Northen, M.D., whose work with soils is quoted in this same Government document, was asked to explain his intense interest in soil minerals. Dr. Northen answered, "I'm an M.D., my work lies in the field of biochemistry and nutrition. I gave up medicine because this is a wider and more important work. Sick soils mean sick plants, sick animals, sick people. Physical, mental and moral fitness depends largely upon an ample supply and a proper proportion of the minerals in our foods."

One researcher says, "There are at least 16 minerals your body needs to maintain good health. They are found in your muscles, brain, glands, heart, hair and blood. You are constantly excreting them and they can only be restored via your diet (or through food supplements). They need to be constantly replenished."

Jonathan Forman, M.D., former editor of the *Ohio State Medical Journal*, adds, "Once Americans begin eating food grown on soil containing all the essential elements, disease will practically vanish, the life span will be about 120 years, childbirth will be painless, and our national disposition will improve."

HOW TO GET MINERALS INTO YOUR DIET

Since we cannot always be sure that the food we buy contains all of the necessary minerals, we have to find other trustworthy sources. Dr. W. A. P. Black, writing in a British magazine, *Agriculture*, says, "Seaweeds have the advantage over land crops in that they grow in an ideal environment in which the nutrients in sea water are constantly being renewed by nature. . . . Seaweeds, therefore, contain all the elements, even vitamins."

There are many kinds of edible and highly nutritious seaweeds available, which we can easily incorporate into our diet in different forms. One of them, Irish moss, is harvested and widely used in New England states for, among other things, a thickening agent for puddings.

Murray Rose, the youngest three-time gold medal winner of the Olympics, made Irish moss, rich in protein, minerals and some vitamins, one of the mainstays of his diet during his training. His nutritionist told me that every day his mother made an Irish moss concoction for him. She took a couple of handfuls of the moss, covered it generously with water, and allowed it to simmer for forty-five minutes. Then she strained it, added concentrated fruit juice, changing the flavor from day to day. She added a bit of honey (a squirt of lemon adds zest, too). Murray loved this dish and ate it every day. Of course it was only a part of his diet, but he felt it was an important part in maintaining his stamina during the Olympics, as he explained in the book *Faith, Love and Seaweed*.*

Here is another Irish moss story. Some time ago a boat loaded with horses was headed toward Ireland. These horses looked at least twenty years old, were sway-backed, with scraggly hair. The boat was shipwrecked. Somehow the horses reached shore and lived only on seafood, mainly Irish moss. When the insurance company located them a year later, they were healthy and beautiful and appeared to be rejuvenated.

Another variety of seaweed, Norwegian kelp, available in this country, has been analyzed and found to contain 11 vitamins, 21 amino acids (proteins), and 60 mineral factors.

One man told me he rubbed a lotion made of Norwegian kelp on several bald spots on his head and new hair began to grow. I felt the new fuzz, myself. There were other witnesses to this change, too. Even more surprising, some of this man's hair, which had previously been gray, came in its original brown. Of course this may not work for everyone, but it's worth a try.

Dulse is still another type of seaweed nutritionally rich. I am told that children who live in Nova Scotia at the Bay of Fundy buy dulse from grocery stores, in ten-cent paper bags, and eat it instead of candy. They have rosy cheeks and look extremely healthy, reporters tell me.

* Englewood Cliffs, N.J.: Prentice-Hall, 1965.

The Japanese are a physically compact, agile, alert, and lean race. One of the main staples of their diet is a seaweed known as *laver*, which they call *nori*. It is pressed into paper-thin sheets, sold in wax-paper bags at Oriental grocery stores, even in America, and nibbled as a snack or used in cooking. A Japanese woman told me that Japanese mothers start giving *nori* to their children at an early age "to keep their hair dark."

Dr. Albert Holand, Jr., says that because it is gelatinous, *nori* can be used as an aid to reducing. He suggests eating it before a meal with a drink of water. It will swell, he says, and thus appease your appetite.

My husband carries a packet of *nori* whenever and wherever he travels. He keeps it in his pocket and between trains and planes takes out a pressed sheet and nibbles it. He swears he feels better as long as he continues to take *nori*. One variety is flavored with soy sauce and sugar, and I must confess I prefer this variety to that which has an undisguised seaweed flavor.

The effect of seaweed has been scientifically tested both on animals and on people, with indisputable good-health results.

GOOD RESULTS FROM SEAWEED

Paul Bragg, an amazing young-old man, is a Tarzanlike species fast disappearing from our civilization. He is fit as a fiddle at eighty-five. He gives credit, in part, for his amazing energy to natural food including seaweed. The *New Zealand Woman's Weekly*, describing his visit to that country, wrote, "How many of us will be setting off for a two-mile run every morning when we're 85? And how many of us, at this same age, will be able to stand on our heads for five minutes, play polo, swim vigorously—and look at least 20 years younger than our age?

"Paul Bragg, of Hollywood, California, has made a business of keeping young and can do all of these things. He is remarkably fit, full of vitality, and bursting with enough energy to make people half his age cringe.

"Mr. Bragg is emphatic that he intends to live to 120— or more. He believes the secret of life is nutrition, and considers there should be university courses to teach people how to eat and what to eat. He chews away at edible seaweed that looks something like red cabbage, dried.

" 'This seaweed,' said Mr. Bragg, 'contains all the 60

nutrients the body requires. In fact we should eat a lot of sea foods.'

"To season his food he uses kelp granules which contain natural salt from the sea as well as other valuable minerals.

"Today he is diet adviser to many stars. 'They pay me to keep them slim, trim and young,' said Mr. Bragg."

Writing in *Let's Live* magazine, Melchior T. Dikkers, Ph.D., a director of a trace mineral research laboratory, describes other good results. He says, "Physicians generally estimate that from 60% to 80% of their patients come to the office suffering from some functional disturbance. This type of patient usually complains of fatigue, memory loss, and difficulty in concentrating. Some individuals become more and more nervous and irritable, developing anxiety symptoms, and become emotional, oftentimes to the point of distress. Others say they have become tired of living. Life is dull and hopeless and they use expressions like, 'What's the use?' or 'I'm tired of it all.'

"Every type of laboratory test made on these patients checks out negative. Their physician states, according to his diagnosis, 'There is nothing wrong with you.' "

Jacques Ménétrier, M.D., director of a biological research laboratory in Geneva, Switzerland, with which Dr. Dikkers is affiliated, has found that trace mineral therapy improves the conditions mentioned above, prevents them from becoming serious, and can eventually return the tissue to normal functioning. Dr. Ménétrier adds that trace element therapy has given good results in the following afflictions:

High blood pressure
Allergies
Premature aging
Resistance to tuberculosis (Myobacterium type)
Flu viruses

During the 1957 Asian flu epidemic, Dr. Ménétrier reports, people who received specific trace minerals were immune to the flu, even though they had been exposed to it.

Henry Picard, M.D., of France, reported that 40 per cent of his patients improved considerably from the use of trace element therapy; 30 per cent showed substantial improvement in arthritic symptoms; there was an increase of freedom of joint movement and a decrease in pain. Thirty per cent showed no improvement; most of these were long-standing cases.

WHY TRACE ELEMENTS IMPROVE HEALTH

Rutgers University found that trace minerals act as catalysts—in other words, they help other minerals and vitamins to be assimilated by the body. Together they make an invincible team. If these trace elements are derived from seaweed there are many elements, known and unknown, that apparently get to work to begin to improve health in many surprising ways. One of the benefits is with colds. For example, a report from an International Seaweed Symposium stated, "In all patients there was a spectacular drop in the incidence of colds. In those colds which were already contracted, the intensity and the duration were so much reduced that the annoyance of the infection was minimal."

This recalls the story of a friend who had employed a Japanese man in his factory. One day the man asked to be excused long enough to go home to get his seaweed. He explained that he was starting to come down with a cold and needed some seaweed quick!

Perhaps one reason seaweeds are so helpful is that they include not only minerals, but vitamins and protein factors as well. Dr. Dikkers, whom I mentioned earlier, says, "Some seaweeds contain more vitamins A and D than cod liver oil. They contain all the B-complex vitamins, vitamin C, and vitamin E. In fact all of the vitamins and minerals are found in larger amounts than in any land vegetation.

"The proportion of minerals is almost identical with that in the human blood. This has been known for years. One wonders why, with all the knowledge available concerning the value of our seaweeds, we haven't used them more abundantly in the past."

Dr. Dikkers lists the following assets of seaweed:

—It has antibiotic qualities.
—It helps to relieve constipation and soothes intestinal irritation.
—It has been used for hundreds of years for diarrhea and dysentery.
—Seaweed extracts were used for the relief of respiratory irritations due to poisonous gas during World War I.

—It has a neutralizing effect on toxic substances, probably due to vitamin C and specific enzymes.

T. J. Lyle, M.D., professor of therapeutics and medicine, states that, though the action of seaweed is slow, it can help the mucous membranes; be a weight reducer; and is valuable in cases of gout, rheumatism, and dropsy.

Eric F. W. Powell, in his booklet, *Kelp, the Health Giver,* adds the following benefits of kelp:

—Aids calcium assimilation.
—Helps nervous disorders.
—Improves arterial disorders.
—Assists a sluggish pancreas.
—Helps the thyroid (and thus fatigue), due to its iodine content.
—Helps the sex glands function, particularly the prostate.

One of the most recently discovered benefits of kelp is that it reduces fall-out in the body. Researchers at McGill University in Canada found that kelp acted as a binding agent or antagonist to Strontium 90. It reduced the absorption of Strontium 90 from 50 per cent to 80 per cent in animals given kelp, whereas the untreated animals did not experience protection at all. The animals which were protected by kelp showed a 75 per cent drop in bone absorption and a 60 per cent drop of Strontium 90 in blood levels. In these days of nuclear testing with resulting fall-out, it is comforting to know that the use of seaweed can give us fall-out protection.

In fact, according to Dr. Dikkers, "The ocean plants contain all of the elements necessary for cell regeneration and repair. Their wonderful healing and soothing properties, for all forms of irritations and inflammations, offer new vistas of possibilities and hope for man's ills in the future."

Since learning the terrific value of seaweeds I have added them in substantial amounts to my own diet. For the most part I take them in tablet form, which I buy at health stores. Whether the seaweed is dried whole, as in Irish moss, dulse, or *nori* sheets used by the Japanese, or in tablets of Norwegian kelp or the Pacific kelp (known by the long name of *Macrocystis pyrifera*), the choice of how you take seaweeds is up to you.

HOW MUCH SEAWEED TO USE

The amount needed for each person has not been settled. Dr. Royal Lee, D.D.S., a nutrition expert, was once asked this question. He answered, "The use of seaweed products depends on the individual need. Since it is a good source of the mineral elements, potassium and iodine, those individuals who are already consuming foods high in these elements would not tolerate or utilize the additional amounts found in kelp. The equivalent of 2 or 3 teaspoons of finely powdered kelp per day is certainly not exceedingly high and would be considered adequate for certain basic mineral support."

Powdered seaweed can be added to liquids such as tomato juice. Kelp tablets are probably easier to take. Two doctors have conducted an exciting study, showing what seaweed has actually accomplished in human health improvement. These doctors are George L. Siefert, M.D., and H. Curtis Wood, M.D., both of Philadelphia. They used Pacific Ocean kelp (*Macrocystis pyrifera*) in tablet form for their patients.

Here is the story in the doctors' own words:

"Four hundred pregnant patients, consecutive cases in private practice, were placed on three mineral tablets a day and their hemoglobin levels were ascertained at each monthly prenatal visit. This series of women started out with an average hemoglobin of 65 per cent, showed a consistent rise each month and after eight to ten weeks of medication they ended up with an average hemoglobin level of 83 per cent. Furthermore, this average rise of 18% units during the pregnancy was accomplished without any of the gastro-intestinal disturbances so often associated with inorganic iron therapy.

"Over the years other patients have reported a great many benefits which they have credited to the minerals used as a food supplement. Time does not permit enlarging upon this aspect of the subject, other than to list a few of them.

—Improvement in the color and quality of the hair.
—Less brittle fingernails.
—Less fragile capillaries, as evidenced by less bruising.
—Relief of certain skin conditions.
—Increase in virility.

—Marked improvement in arthritic cases.
—Relief of eye conditions, such as iritis and cataract.
—Less constipation.
—Increased sense of well-being.

"Conclusion: *Macrocystis pyrifera* is an effective and inexpensive source of trace elements and is useful in human nutrition."

Here is the true story of the effect of minerals on the health of one woman. Her name and the names of two M.D.s confirming her improvement are in my files.

A Case History

About thirteen years ago, at the age of seventy-two, I developed pain and severe swelling in the joints of my body. As the condition became progressively worse I put myself under the care of two medical doctors. Various medical treatments were taken, mainly cortisone, but the condition continued to worsen.

I was told that I had four kinds of arthritis, including Rheumatoid, and nothing could be done beyond the treatment I was receiving. I became almost a total cripple; I could hardly dress myself, comb my hair or do the general house-work. To get around at all it was necessary for me to use two canes. The pain was excruciating!!

I heard of a seaweed product and decided to try it even though I had little hope that I could be helped. In a few weeks I began to feel better. Gradually the pain lessened, my joints freed again and the swelling and fever disappeared and my health began improving.

Today at the age of eighty-four I am very active for my age; I dress myself, comb my own hair, do all my own house-work and shopping, crochet and write letters again.

The doctors are astonished at my excellent health and tell me I am getting younger. Needless to say I cannot praise this seaweed product and supplementary vitamins (later vitamin E and vitamin C were added to the program) enough!!

I do hope other people will be able to profit by my experience.

Sincerely yours,
Mrs. C. H.
Modesto, California

10 Wonder Foods
   Are Wonderful

A certain group of foods is called "wonder foods." This does not mean they produce miracles or are a panacea; no single food is a cure-all. The term merely indicates that, ounce for ounce, these special foods contain more repair materials than others. Laboratory analysis confirms this statement.

People who use them report quicker health benefits than from eating ordinary foods. Since they contain a higher-than-average amount of vitamins and minerals and are surprisingly inexpensive, they are an excellent value. If you were to buy separately the same amount of vitamins and minerals which they contain, your budget would be considerably strained. Furthermore, because these foods are so concentrated in repair materials, you can eat less and derive more nourishment from them. Thus they can prevent a weight gain and a pocketbook loss.

For some reason, much fun has been poked at these special foods, and people who eat them are often labeled "health nuts," "quacks," and "faddists." This concerns me not at all. I, and thousands of others, eat them constantly and thrive on them. We would rather eat nutritionally rich foods and be well, than eat impoverished foods and be sick. For this reason I, for one, am proud to be a healthy "nut."

What are these wonder foods? They include liver, brewers yeast, rice polishings, blackstrap molasses, wheat germ, yogurt, lecithin, various seeds and oils. Keep an open mind until after you have read some of the laboratory analyses (which don't lie). Note some of their excellent health results reported by doctors and laymen. I hope you will agree that these precious foods are truly wonder foods and are well worth incorporating into your own and your family's diet. Here are the values of some of them.

LIVER

Liver probably contains more nutritional values than any other single food. It is a rich source of vitamins, minerals, and easily assimilated protein. For years doctors have prescribed liver in some form as a tonic for those people who are "run down." Liver injections or an oral extract of liver are also used for anemia, since liver contains a rich supply of vitamin B-12. Most doctors and nutritionists recommend eating liver at least once or twice weekly.

You may not like liver. If so, you are not alone. I don't either. Instead, I take desiccated liver tablets. Desiccated liver is whole liver, minus connective tissue and fat, dried at an extremely low temperature so as to conserve optimum nutritional content. The final product is sold in powder, tablet, or capsule form. The nutritional value of desiccated liver ranks second to fresh liver. It is easy to take and effective.

Why is liver so valuable? It is a storehouse of vitamins and minerals. Here is an analysis:*

Analysis of Liver

100 grams of fresh liver (approximately 4 ounces, or an average slice) contains:

Calcium	8 mg.
Phosphorus	486 mg.
Iron	7.8 mg. (hamburger contains only 2.8)
Vitamin A	53,500 I.U. (hamburger contains none)
Vitamin B-1	.26 mg. (hamburger contains .08)
Vitamin B-2	3.96 mg. (hamburger contains 1.19)
Nicotinic acid (another B vitamin)	14.8 mg. (hamburger contains 4.8)
Vitamin C	31 mg. (hamburger contains none)

The vitamin B-12 content is not listed here, or in

* From *Heinz Nutrition Data*, fifth ed., 1964; published by Heinz International Research Center.

Department of Agriculture tables. However, according to another source, the same amount of liver contains 35–50 micrograms of B-12, whereas hamburger contains only 2–5 micrograms.*

There is one caution to keep in mind when taking liver. The liver is not only a depot for storage of vitamins and minerals; it is also a filter for poisons which may enter the body.

One physician who was prescribing liver to his patients suddenly realized that animal liver could also absorb and store dangerous insecticides, some of the very substances he was attempting to eliminate in his patients. For this reason he now supervises the source of his supply of liver. It comes from organically fed animals only and thus is not exposed to insecticides. One large commercial firm, which specializes in producing natural vitamins, derives all of its liver supply for desiccated liver from a South American country where sprays are not used.

There are many advantages of taking liver. One of them is that it supplies energy and outwits fatigue. B. H. Ershoff, M.D., tested desiccated liver as an antifatigue factor with three groups of rats. The first two groups were fed a good diet plus various vitamins. The third group was the only one to receive desiccated liver. In performance tests the first two groups exhibited various degrees of fatigue. The third group, given desiccated liver during the same test, did not get tired at all.

Morton S. Biskind, M.D., considers liver, in addition to vitamins, a necessity for regaining health. He says, "Simply adding desiccated liver or suitable liver fractions to the regime invariably has resulted in a lasting improvement, often evident within a few days."

Liver is useful for beauty, too. A woman with gorgeous skin and hair told me, "I eat lots of liver. It feeds and nourishes my skin and hair from the inside. Before I learned this beauty secret, my skin and hair were drab. Today they are my prized possessions." This woman eats liver often or takes 30 tablets of desiccated liver daily.

Bob Hoffmann, a six-time Olympic coach, recently told me that several of his champions won international titles for weight lifting. "They felt that taking desiccated liver gave them the needed energy to win these titles," Bob said. "After all, this information is not new. It dates back

* Bicknell and Prescott: *The Vitamins in Medicine*, third ed.

to the Ershoff tests with laboratory animals." Bob's
athletes usually take 30 tablets of desiccated liver daily,
but during stiff competition where great energy is needed,
they have been known to take 100 tablets daily.

BREWERS YEAST

Brewers yeast is not a fad food or a new food. Since
the time of the early Greeks and Romans, yeast has been
used for a wide variety of medical purposes. It is generally
used today in dried, nonfermentable form as a type of
nutritional therapy. It is one of the greatest (and cheapest)
sources of B vitamins, minerals, and protein. In fact, if
a shortage of world food continues, it may turn out to be
one of our most important foods. Yeast cells of any kind
grow like mad, as every housewife who has ever used
bakers yeast to make bread or rolls knows. Whereas live
bakers yeast is fed on certain ingredients and kept in a
warm place to encourage rapid multiplication, other yeasts
are fed a different diet, also kept warm, and also multiply
rapidly. As someone has stated, it takes months to grow
an animal for food purposes; it takes only hours to grow
food yeast.

Brewers yeast, a left-over or by-product of beer, is an
excellent source of protein, and comparable to the proteins
in meat and milk. It is much cheaper than animal protein.
The powdered, dried residue, which is "killed" so that it
no longer ferments, becomes the edible product described
in the analysis below. It is literally a gold mine of important nutrients, as the analysis shows. It even contains
gold!

One Brewers Yeast Analysis:

Vitamins	*Amino Acids*	*Minerals*
B-1 (Thiamin)	Lysine	Phosphorus
B-2 (Riboflavin)	Tryptophane	Potassium
B-6 (Pyridoxine)	Histidine	Magnesium
Niacin	Phenylalanine	Silicon
Choline	Leucine	Calcium
Inositol	Methionine	Copper
Pantothenic acid	Valine	Manganese
Para-amino-benzoic	Glycine	Zinc
acid (paba)	Alanine	Aluminum
Biotin	Aspartic acid	Sodium

Vitamins	Amino Acids	Minerals
Folic acid	Glutamic acid	Iron
	Proline	Tin
	Hydroxyproline	Boron
	Tyrosine	Gold
	Cystine	Silver
	Arginine	Nickel
		Cobalt
		Iodine

For a long time brewers yeast was used only for nutritional purposes. Recently, however, due to such a great demand, yeast has been grown primarily as a food crop. This special yeast is called primary grown yeast, or nutritional yeast *(Saccharomyces cerevisiae)*, though the old name "brewers yeast" is still used by many from habit. The analysis for this newer nutritional yeast is often even more potent than brewers yeast. Many dramatic cases of health improvement have resulted from both varieties. People report a pick-up of energy, almost in minutes; relief from fatigue, constipation, nervousness, and indigestion. It is also a perfect reducing food. It is an acceptable protein for vegetarians, too, provided it contains vitamin B-12. Vegetarians who universally suffer from a shortage of vitamin B-12, due to lack of animal protein, are inclined to anemia; therefore they should read yeast labels before buying nutritional yeast, since B-12 does not occur in all yeasts.

ARE ALL TYPES OF YEAST DESIRABLE?

The growth of nutrients in yeast can now be controlled. Some vitamins, such as B-1, can be increased to higher levels. Several nutritionists feel that a balanced proportion of the B vitamins should always be maintained, since too much of one B vitamin in the diet can cause an imbalance of another. This is particularly true of B-1. The ideal solution would be to use a dependable yeast from a dependable company. Even so, every yeast should carry a label stating percentages. One nutritionist believes that the amounts of vitamins B-1, B-2, and B-6 should be the same; that there should be six times as much pantothenic acid, niacin and PABA and 200 times choline and inositol, plus very small amounts of biotin and B-12.

There is one type of yeast, called Torula yeast. Like

plants, which derive their nutrition from the soil in which they are grown, yeasts also derive their nutrition from the medium in which they are grown. August R. Faia, Sc.D. (Hon.), states in *Let's Live* magazine (April 1966), "There are baking yeasts, brewing yeasts, distilling yeasts and wine yeasts. These yeasts must not be confused with 'torula' types of yeast which are grown on waste sulphite liquor from wood pulp used in the manufacture of paper. . . . As with all living things the type and amount of nourishment received has an important relation to health and vitality."

I know an entire family who have long bought and eaten nutritional yeast by the hundred-pound barrel. They have thrived on it. One time, though, for no explainable reason they began suffering from nausea and indigestion. It took much sleuthing to discover the cause. They had changed companies from which they ordered their yeast and they learned that the new yeast, though unlabeled, was torula. When they returned it and resumed eating the original *Saccharomyces cerevisiae* variety, their troubles ceased.

Not all torula is the same. Not all torula is disturbing to all people. Some torula is grown on waste products, is cheaper to produce, and is sold to an unsuspecting public for the same price. Other torula strains may be even superior to the average yeast, as you will soon see. Apparently the difference lies in the food upon which it is grown. In my opinion, the label on yeast should state not only the percentages of vitamin content, but should be required to name these growth-foods media.

In one study conducted at the University of Puerto Rico Medical School, liver necrosis in rats occurred more rapidly if they were deficient in vitamin E. The diets which produced the necrosis contained one type of yeast called yeast-15 or torula yeast-15. Other rats given Anheuser-Busch yeast, Strain G, or several other American yeasts were protected.

In another study reported by a physician at Walter Reed Army Medical Center, rats fed torula yeast as the sole source of protein developed a fatal condition of liver necrosis, whereas those fed cerevisiae yeast remained in good health.

Dr. Conrado F. Asenjo of Puerto Rico, in a panel discussion during a nutrition symposium at Massachusetts Institute of Technology, stated, "Torula yeast protein seemed to be the ideal answer to our country's protein tribulation. Torula yeast is a rich source of protein, . . . but it could be produced locally by using blackstrap molasses, a by-product of our sugar industry, as raw material.

"Not only did torula prove to be low in methionine [an amino acid], but the methionine in it was not effectively utilized. . . . Our human volunteer subjects were seldom able to tolerate more than 15 grams per day without having a gastro-intestinal disturbance."

There is another type of torula yeast imported from Europe which is creating a major sensation. It is a living micro-organism fed on 94 different medicinal herbs which are grown organically without the use of chemical fertilizers or pesticides. It is then combined with honey, malt, and syrup of oranges, and is used as a tonic for people of all ages.

Barbara Cartland, a nutrition reporter, writing in the English magazine *Here's Health,* reports that people who use this European variety of torula say, "I have never felt so well," or "It's like being reborn," or "I feel I can push the world over—I am so full of energy."

"The demand has increased. At first the laboratory in Zürich filled and labelled 6,000 bottles every day. Then it became 16,000 a day. Now 2,500 are completed every hour."

There is at least one strain of torula, widely sold in America, which is also apparently well tolerated. Some others are questionable.

Another European yeast product which is becoming available in this country is a live brewers yeast imported from Germany. It comes in a liquid form, combined with grapefruit juice for safekeeping. It provides live young cells in a medium of natural ascorbic acid (vitamin C). J. Bosse, M.D., of Germany, states, "Side effects of this yeast have never been observed. Fluid brewers yeast is a genuine therapeutic agent, able to shorten treatment of many diseases. Its influence on mental capability was observed in patients of any age."

One woman in Germany, in her eighties, attributed her beautiful, wrinkle-free skin to the use of this yeast.

Dr. Bosse finds that the liquid, live brewers yeast is excellent in strengthening the heart muscle, due to its high protein content and especially to glutathion, which it contains. And because the yeast is also high in orotic acid, a B vitamin, it acts as a liver regenerator.

One other woman who had used this yeast was also interviewed. She had suffered from varicose veins, which her doctor said were inescapable during her pregnancy. Thanks to the liquid, live brewers yeast, the varicose veins cleared up completely, leaving her legs in perfect condition.

The cells in this live yeast have not been killed by heat, as in dried yeast powder, but are treated by a secret process to keep them alive, yet dormant, so that they do not ferment in the body.

When it is combined with bottled beet juice—about 2 to 4 ounces to a bottle capful of the yeast—and served between meals, it makes a very palatable drink. European doctors give it to their patients in a "course" of several weeks or months, followed by an interlude. The course is repeated if necessary. Weight-lifters in this country state that the yeast gives them a decided energy lift.

Although these European yeasts are useful, they are more expensive because they are imported. Our American nutritional yeast in dried form is inexpensive and wonderfully effective.

HEALTH ADVANTAGES OF YEAST

Adelle Davis lists some recent findings of the value of our American nutritional yeast:*

—If the inositol and choline (both B vitamins) content is high, together with liver, wheat germ and lecithin, yeast helps to lower cholesterol.
—In one study, two tablespoons of yeast daily plus a multivitamin capsule, produced a rapid improvement in all 68 people suffering from cirrhosis of the liver. As long as the diet continued, there was no return of liver damage.
—Cases of eczema (also acne) often clear up quickly with nutritional yeast.
—Yeast has greatly increased survival of rats given cancer-causing substances.
—Yeast, plus natural fats, has helped dissolve one-half of the gallstones found in hamsters. The remaining stones were small.
—Yeast has helped to reverse gout.
—The ache and stabbing pains of neuritis are helped with yeast and liver.

* Adelle Davis, *Let's Get Well* (New York: Harcourt, Brace and World, 1965).

In radiation studies at Montefiore Hospital in New York City, cancer patients subjected to heavy radiation and given 3 tablespoons of brewers yeast daily did not suffer from anemia and vomiting, which occurred in patients not protected by yeast.

One woman recently wrote me that her dog developed paralysis in his hindquarters. She added brewers yeast to his diet. His paralysis disappeared and has not returned.

Another woman, writing in *Prevention* magazine (December, 1958), stated: "My husband developed a severe pain in his left jaw. It persisted for days, becoming unbearable. . . . A doctor diagnosed it as *tic douloureux* and knew of no relief for the pain except surgery and morphine. . . . This disease is an inflammation of the fifth nerve of the face. I thought, what is good for nerves? Vitamin B. What is the best source of vitamin B? Brewers yeast.

"That night my husband took two tablespoons of yeast and has had that amount ever since. The results have been almost magic. The pain gradually left. At the end of two weeks it was completely gone and has never returned."

DOES NUTRITIONAL YEAST PRODUCE SIDE EFFECTS?

A relative who was visiting me was envious because I am able to take from 2 to 4 tablespoons of yeast daily. She said, "Yeast gives me energy as nothing else does. But if I take more than a teaspoonful daily it gives me gas."

This is a common complaint and is due to either of two causes: Lack of sufficient intestinal flora, or not enough acid. If the gas is due to insufficient intestinal flora, it will soon correct itself as the yeast is continued. However, in my relative's case, the condition had persisted for over a year. This suggested a lack of hydrochloric acid, necessary to digest the protein. She took home with her some hydrochloric acid-betaine-plus-pepsin, and wrote back enthusiastically, "The HCL did the trick. I can take as much yeast as I want now without being bothered with gas."

HOW TO TAKE NUTRITIONAL YEAST

Yeast can be stirred into liquid, juice or water, and taken between meals. Many people who begin to feel fatigued take a tablespoon or so in liquid immediately instead of coffee and then are rewarded by a return of energy within approximately ten minutes. The good effects last for several hours. Some use it as a reducing food; stirred into liquid and drunk just before a meal it takes the edge off a large appetite and saves eating so many calories.

AVOID LIVE BAKERS YEAST

Many people ask if it is safe to take live bakers yeast. The following answer appeared in Volume 7 of *Developments in Industrial Microbiology*, a publication by the American Institute of Biological Sciences, Wash., D.C., 1966: "For many years, prior to 1948, there was an active campaign to sell live bakers yeast for human consumption, and people were advised by advertisement to mix a cake of yeast with orange or tomato juice as a health measure.

"In 1948, Dr. Parsons of the University of Wisconsin showed that instead of increasing B vitamins in the body, live yeast cells depleted the B vitamins in the intestines because the living yeast cells sequestered the available B vitamins and produced a condition of avitaminosis (loss of vitamins) . . . The sales campaign immediately ceased and since then there has been no sale of live bakers yeast for human consumption."

In brewers or nutritional yeast these live cells are heat-killed, thus are prevented from stealing B vitamins from the body.

YOGURT

Yogurt is not a new food. It has been used for centuries in many European countries and appears regularly on the menus of restaurants there. It is stocked in most supermarkets and in all health stores in America.

The major value of yogurt is that it helps the intestinal tract. It has been found an excellent preventive for constipation and diarrhea, and is often used to nullify the disturbing effects of antibiotic drugs.

When an antibiotic is given, it can kill the desirable as well as the undesirable bacteria in the body. The helpful bacteria tenants the intestinal tract and is known as the intestinal flora. This flora manufactures vitamins B and K, and promotes other intestinal benefits. If the flora is destroyed by antibiotic drugs, indigestion, constipation, and other disturbances may result. European doctors know this and, when prescribing an antibiotic, also prescribe a course of yogurt to prevent the damage.

Yogurt has an added value. It is a natural antibiotic in itself. Studies have shown that an 8-ounce jar, refrigerated for seven days, provides an antibiotic value equal to 14 penicillin units.*

Henry Seneca, M.D., has reported studies in a medical journal showing that yogurt kills amoeba in five minutes; typhus, *S. paratyphus, Br. abortus, V. comma, B. subtillis* in one hour. In two hours it kills *S. pulloran, S. dysenteriae, P. vulgaris, M. pyogenes.* In five hours it kills *E. coli, K. pneumonia,* streptococcus, and staphylococcus. In twenty-four hours it kills *L. lactic, C. diphtheriae, S. mitis,* and *S. fecalis.* Other bacteria too numerous to mention are also destroyed by yogurt. Unlike an antibiotic drug, however, yogurt does away with only the disturbing bacteria, without killing the beneficial bacteria. Truly a wonder food!

Yogurt contains protein as well as calcium, and sufficient acid to help digest both. It is custardlike in consistency, and tastes like buttermilk. Many people have to cultivate a taste for it. Others like it immediately. It is satisfyingly cool on a hot day. After a stomach upset, it is refreshing and healing. At bedtime it promotes sleep, due to its calcium content. Although it is available sweetened and flavored, most yogurt eaters prefer it plain.

Yogurt has even been used as a beauty treatment. One internationally known beauty, writing in *Vogue* magazine, stated that her most valuable beauty secret was an application of yogurt to her face at bedtime, left on overnight. The good effects are easily explained by the protein, calcium, and acid content, beneficial to the skin. It also acts as a bleach.

There are many ways to use yogurt in your diet. You can use it in place of dessert. You can use it as a substitute for sour cream; the thicker varieties have an identical taste and texture but contain less than one-fourth the number of calories. It can be used on baked potatoes (with chives or red caviar) and in salad dressings. It should never be cooked, since cooking destroys its active,

---

* Linda Clark, *Stay Young Longer* (New York: Pyramid Books, 1968).

friendly bacteria. You can buy it, or make your own.*

Yogurt has been called "the educated milk." Keep it in your refrigerator at all times.

BLACKSTRAP MOLASSES

Raw sugar cane is rich in vitamins and minerals. Those who eat this natural product do not develop tooth decay or other health disturbances attributed to refined sugar.

After the sap from sugar cane has been collected, three different products are extracted from it. The first extraction is crystallized raw sugar, which contains some vitamins and minerals. It is later refined into "pure" white sugar, and robbed of all vitamins and minerals. If you wish to use raw sugar as a substitute for white sugar, read your labels.

One health organization has this to say:

"Back in 1947 it became illegal to import the old-fashioned 'raw' sugar due to unsanitary shipping conditions, contamination & lack of uniformity. The public demanded raw sugar. Under the 'trade name,' KLEEN RAW, they produced a sugar by spraying molasses on refined white sugar to make it appear raw. Drop a spoonful of this sugar into a glass of warm water & watch the outside crystals melt away to leave a white sugar sediment. They also make Yellow D sugar, which is a rich brown sugar made from cane-molasses & contains the natural nutrients of vitamins & minerals. Golden C sugar is also from molasses & is further refined, making it lighter. These last two are not as sweet as white or Kleen Raw, thus more is needed in cooking. White sugar is a pure carbohydrate, & contains NO nutrients other than empty calories. They do not color brown sugar . . . the color is from the molasses. The mineral content of the sugars are: 1.0% for Kleen Raw; 2.7% for Golden C and 2.9% for Yellow D. Nature's own unprocessed raw honey is still better than raw sugar." (*Organicville Consumer Report*, Aug. 22, 1967.)

The second extraction produces a light molasses. This may contain more vitamins and minerals than the raw sugar.

The third and final extraction is blackstrap molasses, the nutritionally richest of all three extractions. It is one

* See recipe in Linda Clark, *Stay Young Longer, op. cit.*

of the foods highest in iron. (Iron in one tablespoon of blackstrap is the equivalent to that in nine eggs.) Blackstrap is richer in copper than most foods: It is an excellent source of B vitamins, and contains one of the highest levels of the mineral potassium to be found in *any* food. It contains more calcium than milk. As proof of its nutritional value, here is an analysis of blackstrap molasses from the *Journal of the American Medical Association* (July 14, 1951):

Analysis of Blackstrap Molasses

Five tablespoons of blackstrap molasses contain:

Calcium	258 mg.
Phosphorus	30 mg.
Iron	7.97 mg.
Copper	1.93 mg.
Potassium	1500 mg.
B vitamins:	
Inositol	150 mg.
Thiamin	245 mg.
Riboflavin	240 mg.
Niacin	4 mg.
Pyridoxine	270 mg.
Pantothenic acid	260 mg.
Biotin	16 mg.

The benefits of blackstrap are many.* It is a good laxative. You will see in later chapters where it has been used as a factor in naturally recoloring hair, as well as in reversing hair damage due to permanent waving. Because it contains a large amount of inositol, a B vitamin, it is credited with stopping falling hair. Because it is so high in potassium, it becomes a valuable aid for hearts (Hans Selye, M.D., found that serious heart disease appeared in all of his test animals subjected to stress, except those given potassium or magnesium). Because it contains a higher amount of calcium than milk, it has value for those who suffer from calcium deficiency. Because it is rich in iron, and also copper which helps to assimilate iron, it is beneficial to anemia. It contains practically no sugar, which is in its favor.

Blackstrap molasses can be used in many ways: for cooking; added to yogurt; used in hot water as a tea or in milk as a "milk shake."

---

* See Linda Clark, *Stay Young Longer, op. cit.*

There is one caution to observe. Even though you may enjoy the flavor of blackstrap, do not take it straight. Any sticky substance, no matter how helpful, can erode tooth enamel. Take your blackstrap in liquid form. Rinse your mouth afterward.

Blackstrap is, perhaps, one of the most wonderful of all the "wonder foods."

WHEAT GERM

Wheat germ is a *superior* food. According to the 1950–51 U.S. *Yearbook of Agriculture,* "A grain of wheat, like all seeds, contains the nutriment needed for germination and growth of the seedling. Protein, minerals, B vitamins, fat, and carbohydrates are present in the right proportion for the new plant. . . . The germ or embryo contains a large proportion of the vitamins, and protein of superior quality.

"White flour, as it is milled today . . . has removed the germ, also the greater part of the minerals and vitamins and much of the protein."

The 1959 U.S. *Yearbook of Agriculture* adds, "Losses in milling are even higher for some less familiar nutrients. For example, vitamin E is present in high concentrations in the oil of the wheat germ. Nearly all of this vitamin is removed with the germ."

The United States is rated first in heart disease among all countries in the world. It also is the largest user of white bread and white flour, deprived of wheat germ which contains vitamin E. Why is wheat germ removed? Because it is so delicate; it spoils if left long on the grocer's shelf. So it is taken out entirely and not restored.

Is there any connection between the removal of wheat germ and the high rate of heart disease in the United States? The Minnesota Agricultural Experiment Station found that cattle, though they appeared healthy, suddenly dropped dead of heart disease. The cause was found: wheat germ had been removed from feed rations. When it was restored, the deaths from heart disease ceased.

Vitamin E, found in wheat germ, has been found protective to the human heart by an increasing number of doctors throughout the entire world, though the United States was the last to admit it. Yet our Food and Drug Administration claimed for years that this vitamin was useless. Finally, they had to back down in the face of so much proof to the contrary. Labels on vitamin E bottles are now allowed to state that vitamin E, derived from wheat germ, is necessary in human nutrition.

Vitamin E is concentrated from wheat germ. It provides oxygen to the heart and other muscles. A researcher at the University of Pennsylvania reported almost unbelievable improvement in the heart of chickens fed wheat germ, as compared to those which were denied it.

Wheat germ given regularly may protect humans against heart disease. If heart disease has already threatened, however, additional vitamin E is a wise precaution. Physicians specializing in its use have returned heart patients with serious heart disease to normal activity through large amounts of vitamin E alone. No nitroglycerine or digitalis was added. Victims of heart attacks have been returned to work, even to mowing lawns, as a result of vitamin E therapy by the Doctors Shute in Canada.

Wheat germ oil has been tested by various laboratories on animals, humans, and particularly on athletes, and found helpful in outwitting fatigue. One teaspoon daily was found sufficient to raise the oxygen of the heart to the equivalent of that provided by an oxygen tent.

A three-year university experiment with 500 people showed that wheat germ oil helps heart action and increases endurance.

In addition to vitamin E, wheat germ contains calcium, phosphorus, and B vitamins. One-half cup of wheat germ equals 24 grams of protein, the equivalent of four eggs.

Wheat germ is easy to include in your diet. The toasted variety, vacuum-packed, can be sprinkled on other cereals or floated on top of milk as a cereal in itself. Children love it. It is far more nutritious than the refined cereals heralded by loud commercials as being "high in protein," which they are not.

Wheat germ can be added in baking without altering the flavor. It can be used in biscuits, muffins, breads, waffles, hot cakes, and meat loaves. It can also be used instead of bread crumbs for breading meat and vegetables.

Be sure to keep wheat germ, and wheat germ oil, refrigerated to prevent rancidity.

Analysis of Wheat Germ

Vitamin B-1	.45 mg. per oz.
Vitamin B-2	.14 mg. per oz.

Nicotinic acid	.5 mg. per oz.
Vitamin B-6	.45 mg. per oz.
Vitamin E	7 mg. per oz.
Oil	8.4%
Protein	23%
Copper	.4 mg. per oz.
Iron	2.5 mg. per oz.
Manganese	4 mg. per oz.

Wheat germ oil plays a part in beauty, too.

Dr. M. O. Garten suggests feeding the fingernails wheat germ oil to make them strong. He suggests warming the oil, kept especially for this purpose and refrigerated after each use. Immerse the fingernails in the warmed oil for three or four minutes. Then remove the excess oil with a dry paper towel and massage nails briskly. Any oil which remains on your fingers can be massaged in the skin on your arms or on your hands.

One man reports that he had liver spots on his back and chest and that they kept getting darker and darker. After applying wheat germ oil every night they faded to the point that they were barely visible.

In a later chapter you will see how wheat germ oil can add "body" to hard-to-manage hair and how vitamin E can aid wrinkles.

Here is an example of a woman whose return to health was aided by wheat germ. Bonnie L. Fisher tells that due to her ignorance of diet she had lost her health, but regained it by changing her diet. While she was searching for the real cause of her illness, she submitted to eighteen operations, thinking each one would correct the problem. Finally, weaker but wiser, she devoted what little energy she had left to studying health from the nutritional stand-point. Learning from a Government Bulletin that germ of wheat spoils in a week after grinding, she and her family began to grind fresh grain into flour and cereals daily. They used the freshly ground grain made into bread or mush, or even ate it raw. They also ate many raw fruits and vegetables.

She said, "We were astonished at the results. In two weeks it was plainly discernible that the whole family were improved in health, and the improvement has continued for the three years since. I, who had practically been an invalid for ten years, prematurely old, losing my memory, and with a chronic cough, have so far recovered as to be stronger than in the 'prime' of my life.

"As soon as I was sure I was improving, I began to consider how I could most quickly get the news to other sufferers."

Bonnie Fisher next went into medical libraries (as I have done) seeking the truth about the connection between food and health. She, and I, found that correct nutrition can improve and maintain health. She is another example showing that it can be done.

SEEDS

Many seeds and nuts are excellent sources of nutrition. They are rich in vitamin E, other vitamins, protein, and minerals. Cooking destroys the valuable growth factor.

Sunflower seeds are delightful as well as nutritious. They are a rich source of protein, are excellent to nibble on between meals to raise energy and stave off hunger. In a radio station where my program appeared, I noticed that, on the installation of a new coffee machine, the employees were drinking more and more coffee and getting more and more irritable. Coffee (like sugar) raises the blood sugar suddenly, providing a temporary burst of energy which soon nose-dives, causing that let-down feeling all over again. This is why office workers, even housewives, have acquired the habit of an all-day "coffee break." They drink one cup after another, seeking that needed "lift." Unfortunately, it becomes a vicious circle, providing only temporary energy, followed by a greater letdown. *This does not happen if protein or fat is taken with coffee.* Both protein and fat provide more lasting energy. There are various ways to supply both. Sunflower seeds are one method.

One day I donated a vacuum-packed can of hulled raw sunflower seeds to the radio station and placed it beside the coffee machine. The employees began nibbling a few with each cup of coffee. Several days later one of the secretaries said, "I had never tasted sunflower seeds before. They are delicious. More important, I usually cave in from weariness at four o'clock. Since I have been eating them, I don't notice a four o'clock slump. My energy continues right through the day."

The other employees began to improve, too. Sunflower

seeds contain both protein and fat, plus a host of vitamins and minerals, as the following analysis proves.

Analysis of Sunflower Seeds (¼ pound)

Minerals

Iron	6.0 mg.
Phosphorus	860.0 mg.
Calcium	57.0 mg.
Iodine	0.07 mg.
Magnesium	347.0 mg.
Potassium	630.0 mg.
Manganese	25 parts per million
Copper	20 parts per million

B Vitamins

B-1 (Thiamin)	212 mg.
B-2 (Riboflavin)	0.28 mg.
Niacin	5.6 mg.
B-6 (Pyridoxine)	1.1 mg.
Para-amino-benzoic acid	62 mg.
Biotin	0.067 mg.
Choline	216.00 mg.
Inositol	147.00 mg.
Folic acid	0.1 mg.
Pantothenic acid	2.2 mg.
Pantothenol	3.5 mg.

Other Vitamins

Vitamin D	92 U.S.P. units
Vitamin E	31 Int. units
Protein	25%
Sunflower oil	48.44% (over 90% unsaturated acids)
Ash	3.64%
Crude fiber	2.47%
Carbohydrate	15.18%
Moisture	5.27%

I carry sunflower seeds in my purse when I travel. They have saved me from hunger many a time when food was not available due to a delayed train or plane. Many mothers use sunflower seeds for children's snacks. The seeds can be added to salads, used for toppings on cereals, ice cream, and puddings. Some serve them as nibbles at cocktail time. They are available at health stores and provide a lot of nutrition for the money.

SPROUTED SEEDS

One of the best sources of free vitamins and minerals is sprouts. A physician with four children lived next door to a friend of mine who always kept a bowl of "sprouties" on the table for his children and their friends. Eventually the physician and his family moved away. He wrote, "As long as we lived next door to you, my children stayed in excellent health. Since we have moved, their health is not as good. As I tried to analyze why, the only change I can put my finger on is that they no longer eat the sprouts that you so generously provided. We are going to make them a habit in this family from now on."

Sprouts are inexpensive, simple to grow, and easy to prepare. When seeds are sprouted the various vitamin content increases 10, 50, 100, 500, 600, and even over 1,000 per cent!* Sprouts are especially rich in vitamins B, C, and E. For people who cannot garden, or for those who want a method of easy indoor winter gardening, sprouts are the answer. They can be germinated from any whole, unhulled seeds or beans. The most popular are mung, soy, alfalfa, and wheat.

Since many seeds these days are dipped in deadly fungicides, it is safer to get them from health stores than from seed stores. To prepare them, put a few seeds between paper towels, in a colander. Hold under running water in the sink for a few moments until the towels are thoroughly damp. After draining, put the colander out of the way in a corner of the kitchen counter. Dampen each day, in the same way. Within a few days the seeds will develop little "tails" or sprouts. When they are approximately an inch long, refrigerate them for eating, and start a new batch.

They can be added to salads, sandwiches, or dropped at the last minute (so they won't cook and thus destroy the precious vitamin content) into casseroles, soups, or omelets.

The Chinese, who use bean sprouts daily, have known of their value and flavor for centuries. We are just beginning to catch up with them.

* See Linda Clark, *Stay Young Longer, op. cit.*

LECITHIN

Lecithin, pronounced *less-i-thin*, is found in every cell of the body, and needs to be replaced constantly. It acts as a natural tranquilizer, distributes body weight more evenly, helps to plump up the skin, and, most important of all, reduces cholesterol.*

Lecithin is found in many unprocessed vegetable oils. It is removed in the hydrogenation process, thereby explaining why unsaturated fats have been reported to lower cholesterol levels, whereas saturated or hydrogenated fats apparently raise it.

Lecithin granules are made of soybeans. They look a bit like gelatin, are relatively tasteless, and work wonders. Lecithin is also available in liquid form.

Hans W. Wohlgemuth is chief chemist of the California plant of an international food and beverage company. He studied chemistry in Austria, and came to America in 1951. In 1957 he became research assistant at Ohio State University; then he moved to California and his present position. He tells how he accidentally discovered the beneficial effects of lecithin on health.

He writes, "In my research, I have found that lecithin can be very beneficial to health. But I did not learn this for many years, although I work with lecithin constantly.

"At the chocolate plant where I work, we use lecithin by the ton as an emulsifier.

"As I said, I didn't think much about lecithin until one evening at home, while I was cleaning up my desk. I ran across a little booklet called *Lecithin and Health,* by Edward R. Hewitt.** It is only twenty pages long, but on these twenty pages there is more information about general health which shows more clearly what natural substances can do for well-being than in most heavy volumes I have read. Physicians who have carried out research on lecithin are mentioned in the book.

"One of the chapters is on hardening of the arteries. The book mentions physicians who have learned from their research that lecithin is apparently able to soften and ac-

* See Linda Clark, *Stay Young Longer, op. cit.*
** Published by the Health Publishing Company, 1957, 2126 34th Avenue, San Francisco, California. Available at health stores.

tually rinse away solidified cholesterol which has been deposited on the walls of the arteries. According to this research, cholesterol blood levels have dropped, blood pressure has been lowered, and heart attacks have been prevented.

"I can explain, from my knowledge of the industrial uses of lecithin, why this is true. Sometimes, when we find our chocolate mass too thick, and we already have enough fat content in it, we don't want to add butter to make it thinner. So, instead of adding 80 pounds of butter, we add three pounds of lecithin to thin the consistency. This is industrial proof how the fat, already present, is moved or liquefied by a small addition of lecithin.

"Since we do not ordinarily eat many foods containing much lecithin, and our blood is short of it, the cholesterol is not moved through our system, but is deposited on the walls of the arteries, instead. But if we do have sufficient lecithin, it keeps the cholesterol in solution or in a liquid state, and the arteries are kept free and elastic. Otherwise, the deposits build up, become hard, and the arteries become inflexible like a steel pipe. The blood pressure may rise, and as the arteries become choked with deposits, the pathway may eventually become completely blocked. If this happens, it produces a coronary occlusion, better known as a heart attack.

"The most common source of lecithin is the soybean. We find lecithin in health stores in three forms: liquid, granules, and powder.

"Drying the lecithin produces granules or powder (from which oil is removed). I, personally, prefer liquid lecithin because you can dissolve a hardened oil with another oil better than with a solid.

"Liquid lecithin will keep indefinitely, will not become rancid, and you need never throw it away. It may form a skin or membrane on the top which protects it from the air, and which is dissolved easily by stirring or heating.

"Lecithin is a food. It is not a drug. There is no danger in taking it.

"Lecithin is found in every cell of the human body. Approximately 17 to 20 per cent of our brain is lecithin. Lecithin is high in phosphorus. There is an old German saying, 'No phosphorus, no brains.' Normal brain tissue is thus high in phosphorus, but if an individual's brain is short of phosphoric acid, because it becomes depleted and is not replenished, then even if he is intelligent, his brain may not function, nor will he think or reason properly.

"In addition to the high concentration of lecithin in the brain, it also occurs in the myelin sheath which surrounds the nerves; in the heart, the bone marrow, the kidneys, liver, spinal cord, the blood; and it is necessary for the proper function of the glands, including the sex glands.

"After I learned how important lecithin was to health, I began to experiment to see if there might not be some pleasant way to take it, and I finally found how: by the use of a marmalade.

"To make this marmalade, I chop up a whole lemon—skin, seeds and all—in a blender. (This supplies the missing vitamin C as well as a fruity flavor.) Next I add twice as much honey and three times as much liquid lecithin, mixing it all very well in the blender. This formula is a 1–2–3 ratio: one part whole lemon, two parts honey, three parts liquid lecithin. [Editor's Note: I tried this and, though delicious, found it a little too sweet for some of us who preferred one part lemon, one part honey and three parts of liquid lecithin.]

"This marmalade can be stored in the refrigerator and used on toast, or eaten from the spoon (although it still clings to the roof of the mouth).

"I have found that by using a tablespoon of this mixture night and morning, it supplies at least one teaspoon of lecithin every eight hours and keeps it in the blood stream at all times. Healthwise, one should not expect results in less than two months.

"I began to give this marmalade to my friends. One man worked in a shop where I had gone to have a sieve soldered. He was a nervous wreck and his hand shook like a leaf. I suggested using the marmalade. After four to six weeks, his hand was still not quite steady but it was much better. He also looked better.

"I had another friend who was very ill with myasthenia gravis. This is a paralysis of the muscles. He had been in a wheel chair for years and could not even keep his eyelids open.

"Learning that lecithin is good for the muscles, and wanting to help this poor man if possible, I asked him if he would be willing to try the lecithin marmalade. He agreed, and I went to see him every week.

"After about four weeks, I noticed he began to have a little color in his cheeks. That was the first sign of improvement. After two months, he could lift his arms. It took six months for him to walk up the aisle to the altar at church, with a cane, to take communion. Today, he is playing golf.

"Now is this a miracle? He no longer lives in my area, but last Sunday he came back to visit the church. When he saw me, he said, 'I am still taking lecithin!'

"Mr. Hewitt, in his book, says, 'I have observed where mental ills were greatly improved or entirely cured by lecithin. If the lecithin did actually effect these cures, it is conceivable that it furnished the cell-making material which was previously deficient in the brain cell.'

"He continues, 'Dr. Dietrick of El Paso, Texas, has treated many cases of diabetes with lecithin and reported that the insulin requirement is lessened.'

"He adds, 'If arthritis is due to cholesterol deposits, as some seems to be, lecithin should be helpful.

" 'However, one has to be careful. Lecithin is not a panacea. It will not cure all cases of hardening of the arteries or coronary troubles or diabetes or arthritis, because these diseases can have several causes. It depends on what the real cause is.'

"A recent benefit of lecithin was announced by *Medical World News*, May 17, 1968, which reported 'Lecithin, an emulsifying agent used to keep chocolate smooth and fresh, may also be helpful in preventing gallstones. The reason: lecithin is important in keeping bile cholesterol in solution, and because some gallstones are made of cholesterol coming from the bile, added lecithin might prevent their formation.'

"Lecithin does not have the general approval of the AMA. I have asked doctors—family doctors, friends and others—about their opinion of lecithin. I learned that it was not well known to most doctors.

"Since Nature works slowly to produce benefits, and lecithin is a natural substance, it takes time; not a day or two, but anywhere from three to six months to a year. The doctors told me their patients were just not willing to wait that long for benefits.

"Again let me remind you why lecithin works. Mr. Hewitt says, 'It must be well understood that lecithin is not a drug in itself. It simply furnishes some of the materials that the body needs for growth and renewal of cells. . . . I myself regard it as a dietary essential and feel that by furnishing necessary materials for cell renewal it will increase the length of the active healthy human life.' "

In the next chapter I will tell you about a man who made himself over, with lecithin playing the key role. Meanwhile, incorporate as many "wonder foods" into your diet as possible. You will be rewarded by results.

11 What about Doctors?

One of the questions asked me over and over again is: "Where can I find a nutritionally trained doctor?"

I have a *very* short list of doctors in the United States who use nutritional therapy. There is a tremendous need for thousands more. These nutritional physicians tell me that they have discovered the wonderful effects of nutritional therapy after they left medical school and have consequently trained themselves. As a result of using such therapy their success has soared. By word of mouth one patient tells another how his condition has been alleviated or reversed without pain, hospitalization, drugs, or great expense. Furthermore, the good response is permanent as long as the patient continues the nutritional technique. I predict that the day will come when all doctors will use this method. By so doing, they will prevent most illness and help people to maintain health. In China, for centuries patients have paid their doctors as long as they remained well. They have stopped paying them when they become ill. This is the goal for which we should aim in the United States.

Many doctors, like most people, believe the misrepresentation that nutritional treatment is faddish or quackish. They are also afraid their practice will fall off if they shift to another method of treatment. Nothing could be further from the truth. Many patients are becoming fed up with dangerous and temporary drug treatment. They are becoming alarmed by unnecessary surgery, endless laboratory tests, and multiplying hospital costs. They realize that doctors themselves are also dying of the same diseases they are trying to cure in their patients. The present method of "Doctor, heal thyself" is apparently not working for them any better than for their patients. Hence their image is slipping. Something must be wrong. It is: the average physician is still relying upon the old method of trying to *patch up* his patients so they will hold together a while longer, instead of eliminating illness and building lasting health.

In support of this concept, Dr. Halbert L. Dunn, chief of the National Office of Vital Statistics, stated, "We are interested in defects only. It's like putting patches on tires, and we are getting rapidly to the point where patching is too difficult."

Jonathan Forman, M.D., agrees. He says, "American medicine exists for the care of the sick. It has little or nothing to do with health. . . . We must stop promoting sickness and protect our health."

ARE WE REALLY HEALTHY?

A 1962 issue of a medical magazine, *Clinical Physiology*, states, "The people of the United States are not a well people. Two out of three of them are victims of a chronic disease or a physical handicap. Consequently it takes over 18,000,000 pounds of aspirin, 1,000,000 pounds of barbiturates [sedatives], 800,000 pounds of tranquilizers, astronomical amounts of caffeine, alcohol and nicotine to keep them going." These conditions reported in 1962 are even worse today.

Herbert Ratner, M.D., adds, "America is the most over-medicated, most over-operated and most anxiety ridden country in the world—yet one of the unhealthiest countries in the world. We are flabby, overweight, have a lot of dental caries [cavities] fluoridation notwithstanding. Our gastrointestinal system operates like a sputtering gas engine. We can't sleep; we can't get going when we are awake. We have neuroses; we have high blood pressure. Neither our hearts nor our heads last as long as they should. Coronary disease at the peak of life has hit epidemic proportions. Suicide is one of the leading causes of death between the ages of 15 and 44. We suffer from a plethora of the diseases of civilization."

Cecilia Rosenfeld, M.D., though admitting realistically that not all diseases have their origin in poor nutrition, says, "There is abundant scientific evidence which suggests that many diseases of advancing age such as arthritis, abnormal heart conditions, arteriosclerosis, high blood pressure and other diseases, do not mysteriously begin late in life but have their origin in the bodies of the young people who have not received correct nutritional guidance."

Henry Trautman, M.D., is even more blunt. He says, "Underlying all disease in this artificial world of today is the high incidence of nutritional deficiency. Some authorities estimate the frequency of deficiency as high as 90%. Others agree with Cavanaugh of Cornell University who says, 'There is only one major disease and that is malnutrition. All other ailments to which man is heir are results of this one major disease.'"

Even the influential *Journal of the American Medical Association* (March, 1963) has admitted, "Medical education and medical practice have not kept abreast of the tremendous advances in nutritional knowledge."

WHY IS NOTHING DONE?

A very small percentage of enlightened scientists and physicians are trying to turn the tide in the right direction. The trouble is that there are so few of them that they need the help of the public to succeed. Scientists at the Nobel Institute in Sweden have begun a search for the type of nutrition which will prevent illness and provide physical and mental strength. It is the first time that such an influential group has publicly announced that proper nutrition can achieve health and prevent illness.

In America there are a few hopeful signs. In spite of the fact that the value of nutrition is usually dismissed in this country as faddism, there are some who have learned differently.

For example, one physician, whom I know and admire, told me his story of how he began using nutritional therapy. He had graduated from a well-known midwest medical school and had later specialized in dermatology (skin diseases). He had never heard of the effects of nutrition on health until he married a nutritionist. He became so intrigued with his wife's nutritional experiments on animal health that one day he gathered up his courage and decided he would try nutrition on several of his patients. To his amazement, not only did their skin disturbances completely disappear, but other ailments as well. With great excitement he began using the nutritional approach on more and more patients. He also began to hunt for, and read, every word he could find on the subject of nutritional therapy.

Gradually this physician used fewer drugs and more nutritional substances, until today he uses nutritional therapy exclusively. Did his practice fall off, as many physicians fear? Decidedly not! This man is so busy he has no time to answer the phone (except in emergency) or hundreds of letters, either as a result of his delighted patients or because of articles he has written for medical journals.

This physician now has in his office a huge filing wheel, electrically operated. By stepping on a pedal he can turn to, and stop at, scientific reports of nutritional therapy for every disease. The information contained in this unique and easily available file is kept up-to-date weekly, a giant task in itself, considering the amount of mushrooming nutritional literature now becoming available.

The introduction of another M.D., whom I know, to the exciting world of nutrition came about because his prized dogs, one after another, even though presumably well-fed, suffered from a form of paralysis. Someone suggested changing the dogs' nutrition. The corresponding improvement so impressed the physician that he made a change in his own and his family's nutrition. Here he met with such success that he began applying it to his patients. Today he, too, has given up the use of drugs and has incorporated nutritional therapy exclusively. His practice has also grown by leaps and bounds as his patients' health improves and they tell others about it.

So the news is slowly traveling. A group of 128 physicians and dentists, together with their wives, decided to volunteer as human guinea pigs to see what nutrition could do for their own health. All of this self-experimental group have the results of their blood-chemical analysis and medical histories on computer punch cards. For two years they will keep records of what they eat and the course of their health. Those with specific ailments, including teeth, eyes, nerves or respiratory systems, will be watching for any change in these disturbances.

They explain why they are taking this unprecedented

step: "Many of us concluded that we know more about sickness and disease and less about health and that our failure in prevention ensues from this general lack of knowledge concerning optimal health. . . . When the nagging questions concerning nutrition arise, the situation is quite clouded. The subject has been poorly taught (and still is) in most medical and dental schools so our background is inadequate."

This concept is shared by a few other doctors. In a medical journal, Robert R. Levin, M.D., wrote, "The science of nutrition has made rapid progress in the past 25 years, but its impact on clinical medicine has been slow. There has been an unaccountable delay in the use of nutritional advances by the practicing physician. Medicine has for so long a time devoted its energies to the detailed study of pathology and disease that it has overlooked the importance of nutrition as an etiological [causative] factor of major significance."

WHAT IS THE SOLUTION?

Whereas, on one hand, dire warnings are being sounded to the American people (and doctors) against the "quackery and faddism" of nutrition, on the other hand the truth is gradually coming to light. Alex J. Linck, D.D.S., puts his finger on the real problem: *Nutrition as a science is not taught in any university in this country. Medicine and dentistry are taught from a remedial, not a preventive standpoint."*

If nutrition were to be taught in medical schools, all doctors would be trained to use this therapy for the prevention of illness and the maintenance of health. To their everlasting credit, there are some pioneers who are trying to change this medical school picture. Pleas for medical school training have been repeatedly made by many nutritionists, outstanding doctors, and scientists from well-known universities.

Even if the project does get off the ground and nutritional training finally does become accepted by medical schools, it will take a long, long time for young doctors to complete their pre-training, actual training, internship and finally begin to practice. Meanwhile many people are suffering and in need of help now. Many of these people will not be living in ten or twenty years, if and when this reform does take place.

The only suggestion I can offer is that you, as a patient, try to encourage your doctor to learn more about nutrition and to begin to use it now. Some doctors maintain a thoroughly closed mind. They have always practiced in a certain manner, acceptable to themselves, and they will continue to do so. They are the ones who will accept without question the misinterpretation of facts that nutrition is "quackery." But there are others who have already experimented with nutrition and undoubtedly noticed improvements in their patients. These doctors should be the most receptive to your requests. After all, they have probably already used a sprinkling of nutritional therapy, such as calcium for pregnant women and injections of vitamin B-12 for pernicious anemia. They do not realize that there is much more they can do. This is where your encouragement can help.

After I began to notice the good results of nutrition in my own case, I gave copies of books on nutrition, and later, my own books, to two of the physicians who had treated me. I asked them to try to squeeze in a few minutes now and then in their busy schedules to read them. The trial proved successful. One of the doctors, who had already been suspicious of the fanfare about every "wonder drug" as it had been rapturously announced, had been cautious about prescribing them until their safety and effectiveness were assured. He turned out to be an excellent candidate for the use of safer nutritional treatment. He read the books and began to apply the knowledge. One day I met him on the street and he said, "You know, I tried vitamin E on a patient whose condition had defied all other treatment, *and it worked!*" He was as excited as a child at Christmas.

The other doctor, a more sedate type, never admitted that he had read or tried the nutritional information, but whenever we met socially, he asked with suppressed excitement, "What is new in nutrition?"

Physicians well know that if their patients don't get results from one doctor, they will often go to another. Therefore they are more susceptible to pleasing you than you may think. If you take not emotionally packed or flamboyant literature (which antagonizes them) but sensible and well-documented information on the subject of nutrition-and-health, perhaps they, too, will become interested in learning about and using more nutritional therapy.

Meanwhile, while you are waiting, you can do what I and many others have done: learn to help yourself.

The length of time in which you can expect to see improvement depends upon the extent of your physical condition and your deficiencies. Children respond almost immediately. Others vary from age to age. One of the best examples of health recovery I have ever witnessed occurred in a handsome, heavyweight wrestling champion. Until the end of his thirties he had exercised constantly in order to maintain his title as champion.

Bob, the champion, decided just before he reached the age of forty to retire from the ring. Then disaster struck. Gradually he began to feel worse. Pain in his joints appeared until it became so excruciating he could scarcely sleep. He went from doctor to doctor seeking help. He was given many drugs, including cortisone, or its derivatives, for arthritis. This did not produce permanent relief and only succeeded in making him moon-faced. But arthritis was not his only complaint. His entire body seemed to break down physically.

Finally, the last doctor he visited pronounced his sentence: six weeks to live.

Shortly afterward he was introduced to a nutritionist who told Bob he thought he could help him. He immediately outlined a program which included not one but every nutrient known. This was a massive attack plan, and it worked. Six weeks later, instead of being dead, Bob was playing golf. True, he was not yet 100 per cent well, but he had turned the corner so dramatically that he knew he was on his way to complete health. It took him approximately two years to become completely pain-free and a vitally healthy person. During this time his hair turned back from gray to its original glossy black; his pallor disappeared, and he became ruddy once more. When he ceased taking cortisone his moon-faced condition disappeared. He looked years younger.

I have colored before-and-after pictures to prove this story, as well as the affidavit of the nutritionist who guided him back to health.

THE MAN WHO MADE HIMSELF OVER

I have talked with another man and checked his story thoroughly. I have the names of the doctors who confirm his improvement. I have talked with people who knew him before as well as after his rehabilitation. Here is the story in his own words:

"At the age of fifty-two I began to have symptoms of shortness of breath. This had been building up for three years but I had been blaming it on bad digestion.

"Gradually severe chest pains developed. I had difficulty in walking fast and climbing stairs. One day in New York City it took me fifteen minutes to climb a flight of subway stairs. A companion was so worried he urged me to see a doctor.

"I complied. The doctor took a cardiogram which showed a condition nearing angina pectoris. Tests showed a high cholesterol and cholesterol plaques. He immediately gave me medication, which he warned I would have to take the rest of my life. He also put me on a fat-free diet. I faithfully followed the diet for a while. Meanwhile I developed osteo-arthritis in my shoulder and neck, which became terribly painful. For seven months I sat upright in a chair and between the heart pains and arthritis pains scarcely slept one full night.

"I went to another specialist. His X-rays showed vast deposits of calcium and degeneration of tissues. I was put into traction and given exercise. The results were almost nil. I could not use my arm and still could not sleep.

"One day a friend loaned me a book on health and nutrition. I decided to study this approach seriously and work out a diet on my own. I began to take, daily, two tablespoons of lecithin granules, two tablespoons of brewers yeast, two tablespoons of cold-pressed oil, two teaspoons of cider vinegar, one tablespoon of linseed oil, all in V-8 juice. I added a few tablespoons of wheat germ to my cold cereal.

"The results were unbelievable. Within three weeks I was climbing four flights of stairs to an apartment where I was visiting, without shortness of breath, chest pain or the fear of a heart seizure.

"I was so encouraged with the effect of nutrition on my heart condition, I decided to tackle my arthritis. This I did by beginning a complete vitamin therapy program. I took vitamin E, B-complex, calcium, magnesium, glutamic acid, choline, inositol, kelp, ascorbic acid (vitamin C), and vitamin A. I took different assortments at each meal: eight in the morning, nine at noon, and eight at night. Again the result was unbelievable.

"In three or four weeks I raised my left arm without pain. I found that I did not have to favor it and it soon became normal. In addition, headaches, which had afflicted me since childhood, became further and further apart. My dentist, who, two months previously, was concerned with my bleeding gums, found them healthy and firm, and my tooth decay was reduced to zero. Heartburn also disappeared.

"I returned to the original doctor who lives in Canada and who had prescribed drugs and a fat-free diet. He was overjoyed at my appearance and condition. He said, 'Well, the drug and diet is working.' I told him I was using neither and I wanted another cholesterol test.

"He argued that it was too soon for another test. I insisted. Finally he agreed. I was in his office a few days later when he called the laboratory for a report. The laboratory said, 'You must have sent a blood specimen from the wrong man; this report doesn't make sense.'

" 'What is the reading?' the doctor asked.

" 'The cholesterol level is 69 points lower, impossible in so short a time.'

"So the doctor took another blood specimen. The laboratory found it was identical with the first reading. The doctor asked in disbelief, 'What on earth have you been doing?'

"I answered, 'I have been improving my nutrition and I have been taking lecithin to lower my cholesterol. Have you ever tried it?'

"The doctor looked a little perplexed. He answered, 'Well I have heard of it but I have never tried it with any patients.' I left.

"I have experienced other benefits on my nutritional regime. My hair has stopped falling. Dandruff has disappeared. I was almost completely gray at fifty-two. My hair has recovered a great deal of the original brown color. My skin is vastly improved, too.

"I have unlimited energy now and a zest for life to which all of my friends will testify. Nutrition literally saved my life."

One of the most amusing true stories I have heard is

that of a doctor's wife who had discovered the benefit of "health foods" such as brewers yeast, wheat germ, yogurt, etc. on her health. After watching her own energy increase on this type of diet plus vitamin-mineral supplements, and her doctor-husband's energy decrease on a regular diet, she laid down the law. "You start eating right and taking vitamins yourself, or else!" she commanded. The doctor obeyed "orders."

A news item from UPI dated October 3, 1968, tells of another doctor deeply interested in nutrition.

NEW YORK—(UPI)—Dr. Victor Heiser, at age 95, looks like his own best example of the health-preserving effects of a well-balanced diet.

The 6-foot-2, slim physician has worked more than 70 years as a public health educator, administrator and researcher.

But he also has a continuing interest in good diet as a means of maintaining health.

"We could empty half the hospitals in the country if we could persuade people to eat a proper diet," he said.

"I once induced a friend of mine who's a surgeon in Chicago not to give his children anything with sugar.

"They never had a cavity until college when they began eating sweets."

Dr. Heiser deplored the tendency of young people to fill up at lunch on hamburgers or a salad, sweet rolls, cake or pie and soft drinks. He blamed the high incidence of bad teeth on high consumption of soft drinks.

Ideally, he'd like to see people cut out all desserts except raw fruit, but conceded that this is unlikely to happen, although berries, apples, oranges, pears and other fresh fruit and vegetables now are available all year.

He believes people could ensure good health by eating whole wheat bread, milk—preferably skimmed—yellow vegetables such as carrots and sweet potatoes plus a general line of vegetables, protein foods—meat, poultry, fish, eggs and cheese, and fresh raw fruits.

Dr. Heiser also advocated thorough chewing of food— "nature can't extract enzymes if the food isn't well-chewed."

Dr. Heiser, a former chief health officer for the Philippines, was with the Rockefeller Foundation for 25 years, until his retirement at the age of 65.

These true stories are being duplicated in hundreds of cases throughout the world. By all means seek the help of a nutritionally enlightened physician—if you can find one.

But if it proves impossible, then follow the example of others in the same boat. Read, study, learn everything you can find on the subject of nutrition and health. And then, *do-it-yourself*. It may not be the ideal way, but it is better than nothing at all.

PART II

BEAUTY

12 How to Have Beautiful Skin

There are two ways to beautify your skin: internally and externally. Let's start with the internal method.

In addition to protein, other nutrients are necessary for skin beauty. Most dermatologists (skin specialists) agree that a balanced diet is a *must;* that no human skin can reach its potential beauty or be beautiful for long without good nutrition.

Irwin I. Lubowe, M.D., writes, "There is no doubt that the kinds and amounts of foods we eat have a profound effect upon the skin.

"Diet is a route by which help can be provided to an aging skin. I frequently find that some element necessary for skin health is missing entirely from the usual diet or is present only in inadequate amounts."*

Diane P. Rashey, writing in *Herald of Health,* sums up the role of the skin, which, she reminds us, lives and breathes and is considered a body organ. She says, "The skin cannot be perfect if any other organ is out of order, especially the colon and liver. Malfunctioning of these organs causes toxins to spread into the blood stream which tries to carry them to the skin for elimination. Besides using proper nutrition, the skin itself must be properly cared for. It must be revitalized and invigorated, for by being overused it loses its firmness and elasticity. Flabbiness and wrinkles come little by little. You should take care of your skin long before the ravages of the years start to show.

"The skin of the face and neck is the first to be affected due to the condition within, because of its eliminative role;

---

* Irwin I. Lubowe, M.D., *New Hope for Your Skin* (New York: E. P. Dutton, 1963).

and from without, because of its constant exposure to the weather.

"Wrinkles are caused by a devitalization of the skin as a result of a deficiency of vital food elements. They are furthered by frowning and other facial grimaces.

"This is why nutritious food, containing *all the elements* needed for regenerating our bodies, is so important. Our wonderful organism draws from these elements the power to rebuild new cells constantly to replace those broken down. What is usually thought to be the result of age, is merely the result of incorrect diet and care of the body and skin. The appearance of poor skin and hair can be considerably delayed, if not prevented, by intelligent and persistent care of both the inside and the outside of the body."

Belle Wood-Comstock, M.D., adds, "The appearance of the skin is often an indication of the state of one's health. Eat the right kind of food to properly nourish the skin. Cleansing the skin and purifying the blood is important for healthy skin, too. For purity of blood one must also breathe fresh pure air, exercise out of doors to thoroughly burn cell wastes. . . .

"Foods which tend to clog the skin are greasy foods, rich desserts, white sugar and candy, white bread."

A nutritionist was discussing beauty problems with a beauty operator, who was telling about his patrons' complaints of brittle nails, enlarged pores, leathery skin, and dry, bristly hair. "Actually," said the beauty operator, "a good many of the beauty problems we try to overcome are in your field—nutrition."

WHAT NUTRIENTS HELP SKIN?

Some natural foods are the basis for successful beauty secrets, known and used for centuries. One of the beauty secrets of English royalty—Queen Elizabeth, the Queen Mother, and Princess Margaret—involves barley. Mrs. Alma McKee, who was chief cook to the royal family for many years, says in her book, *To Set Before a Queen,** "There is one secret which may provide a clue to those flawless complexions—barley water. It was always on the dining table. In fact they drank so much that I felt there must be something in it and tried it myself. A day or two

* Simon & Schuster, 1964.

on barley water is wonderfully purifying . . . does wonders for the skin. The recipe was one I took with me when I left the Royal household and in view of its beneficial effects I hope I shall be forgiven! Here is the recipe:

½ cup pearl barley
2½ quarts boiling water
2 lemons
6 oranges (make sure these have no added coloring or preservatives)
Brown sugar or honey to taste

"Put barley in large saucepan, add the boiling water and simmer at low heat, with the lid on, for one hour. Meanwhile squeeze the fruit and keep the juice. Strain the water from the cooked barley into a bowl and add the sugar (or honey) and rinds from the oranges and lemons. Allow to stand until cold. Remove the rinds and add the orange and lemon juice. Keep in refrigerator."

Silicon is called the "beauty mineral," as it is essential to the growth of luxurious hair and natural sheen. It promotes growth and gives strength to nails. It keeps the skin from becoming flabby, and the eyes bright. The chief sources of silicon are "steel-cut" oats, apples, honey, avocados, artichokes, and sunflower seeds.

Dr. Reginald T. Brain, author of a book on skin diseases, believes that fish oils, brewers yeast, desiccated liver, and rose hips (which contain vitamin-C complex) taken internally can do more for your skin than any *synthetic* surface application.

OILS ARE A MUST

W. A. Krehl, M.D., states, "Several types of skin problems (dryness, scaliness, etc.) eczematous in character, have long been associated with the long-term consumption of diets low in fat. One skin disease, phrynoderma, common in India, has shown that the administration of raw linseed oil or linoleic acid produced marked clinical improvement in two to four weeks and cured many patients in four to twenty-four weeks. Even better results were obtained when pyridoxine (vitamin B-6) was combined with the essential fatty acid."

Natural vegetable oils, available from health stores, are preferable. Unsaturated oils are all helpful to skin and hair and if properly used *will not add weight.* Two tablespoons daily are usually recommended. Take your pick: soy, safflower, corn, sunflower, avocado, or a mixture of them all, are excellent. In any French dressings I add virgin olive oil for extra flavor. You can use these oils in salad dressings. One of the best ways of all to add a sheen to your skin and hair is to take cod liver oil. It contains both vitamins A and D.

This reminds me of an incident in my own family. Three of my grandchildren decided to enter a few of their chickens in the country fair. They ordered a government bulletin which gave tips on judging. One tip advised feeding the chickens cod liver oil to produce glossy feathers. This came as a complete surprise to the children. They had always taken cod liver oil at my insistence, but had done so grudgingly, not because they objected to the flavor (they didn't) but because their friends weren't required to take it.

Now they looked at cod liver oil in a new light. Anxious to win a blue ribbon for their chickens, they dutifully fed them cod liver oil, and sure enough the feathers soon became beautiful and glossy.

The result of this project brought mixed blessings. The children now line up cooperatively at bedtime for their tablespoon of cod liver oil, even though their chickens did not win blue ribbons (their chickens were utility birds or *laying* hens, not *show* birds). But the judge kindly explained that cod liver oil improves the appearance of both.

Another vote for cod liver oil came from a friend who used to live in Chile. She wrote me: "My mother was visiting me from Chile. She brought with her her maid Clema. Now, Clema had a condition on her skin in which her hands were so dry they would break open in long cuts along her fingers, and bleed. Since she washed dishes and clothes constantly, she had been having a terrible time with her hands for years, even though she is only twenty-three years old.

"I suggested that she take cod liver oil. In about three months the condition disappeared and her hands have never been better. She says she will never stop taking it."

I, personally, have seen skin and hair acquire a sheen within two weeks after beginning cod liver oil. I dislike the flavor but this is how I make it palatable—even delicious. I buy the mint-flavored variety and keep it refrigerated. I also buy paper cups and have chilled fresh or frozen orange juice ready. In one little cup I add 1 tablespoon of cold mint-flavored cod liver oil. In the other I add two tablespoons of ice cold orange juice. I toss the two liquids back and forth from cup to cup until well blended, then drink. Try it, and you will be pleasantly surprised at the flavor.

Some investigators believe that if you take cod liver oil at bedtime on an empty stomach, you will not gain weight because the oil does not mix with the food. If you prefer, you may follow the suggestion of a woman M.D. who insists that her patients take four capsules of crude cod liver oil every night at bedtime.

WHAT VITAMINS HELP?

A study by a prominent dermatologist in Japan, Dr. Katsu Takenochi, compared the diets of patients with healthy skins, and others with skin diseases. He found that those with skin diseases were deficient in B vitamins. He stated that while only about 1 per cent of the vitamin B we eat reaches the skin, the health of the skin demands it and these water-soluble vitamins must constantly be replaced for skin health.

Dr. Krehl lists the results in skin and hair of the *lack* of all vitamins:

Vitamin A Deficiency

"Vitamin A deficiency causes dryness, scaliness, scalp abscesses and bleaching, drying out and loss of hair. One type of skin eruption is also due to a vitamin A deficiency. . . . Proper diet causes a gradual improvement. As might be expected, those skin lesions which are associated with a deficient intake of vitamin A respond to therapy with this vitamin."

Aida Grey, a beauty expert, knows that vitamins on the inside hasten outside beauty. She has discovered that a shortage of vitamin A can cause large pores, scaliness, dry rough skin and blemishes. If you are troubled with rough skin and blackheads, you may benefit from using vitamin A. Vitamin A can be added to your diet by green or yellow vegetables or fruits, as well as vitamin A supplements.

Vitamin B-Complex Deficiencies

Dr. Krehl states: "Experimental animal studies in which nearly all of the B-complex vitamins have been established are all associated with some skin or hair changes ranging from mild to severe. Riboflavin, niacin, pyridoxine, and pantothenic acid are the members of the B complex group of vitamins that have clinical dermatological significance for man. Other B vitamins which have been found to affect the skin or hair are inositol, PABA, biotin."

Brewers yeast and liver contain them all.

Adelle Davis believes that lack of any of a dozen vitamins can cause eczema or dermatitis and that a completely adequate diet is necessary to ensure the health of the skin. Vitamins A and E, the B-complex group, vitamin C, and minerals are all involved. Adelle states that vitamin C—at least 100 mg. of ascorbic acid taken with each meal —has helped skin abnormalities resulting from allergies and speeds healing. She adds, "Severe eczemas have been treated successfully by 6 heaping tablespoons of brewers yeast daily. I have never seen a case of eczema which did not clear up after getting large amounts of the B vitamins from natural sources."

Dr. Paul Kline of New York City considers vitamin B one of the "musts" for acne. He also administers vitamin A. Dr. Kline treated twenty-five patients with vitamins A and B for eight months and only one failed to show improvement.

Dr. Jon V. Straumfjord treated 100 of his acne patients with large doses of vitamin A. He gave no medicine and no special ointment. Thirty-six patients were completely cured; forty-three were cured except for an occasional pimple.

I know three teenage boys who formerly suffered from acne. They drink their brewers-yeast-and-juice faithfully every morning, eat natural foods, and take their vitamins (they use both A and C). After their skin cleared, wild horses couldn't get them to go back to the diet of the other teenagers: soft drinks, sweets, potato chips, etc.

Vitamin C Deficiency

Dr. Krehl says: "In vitamin C deficiency there is impairment of the structure of the ground substance of the connective tissue."

One type of skin disturbance was nutritionally cured by a wise doctor. His patient, an elderly man, had tried all sorts of creams and ointments without success for three years. Finally, his doctor told him he would have to cure the condition from the *inside*. When he started taking vitamin C, wheat germ oil capsules, and wheat germ on his cereal, the condition completely cleared up.

Aida Grey believes that vitamin C strengthens the tissue underlying the skin, making it firmer.

Vitamin E Deficiency

Vitamin E stimulates fresh oxygen to the tissues. It is found in wheat germ and wheat germ oil: it comes in concentrated form in capsules. Aida Grey, beauty consultant, has found that oxygen helps to repair damaged cells. She says it can help tired skin look fresher within two hours.

Adelle Davis has reported that when she has pierced vitamin E capsules and squeezed the contents onto the scars produced by burns, the scars disappeared.

A SURPRISING NEW BEAUTY TREATMENT

The use of vitamin E on scars led to a most exciting last minute beauty discovery. Just before it was time for this book to go to press, a friend told me that an aged woman had acquired a serious skin disease on one side of her face. The doctors pronounced the condition hopeless. Her son, after reading of the effect of rubbing vitamin E on the skin to remove scars, decided to try it on his mother's face.

Twice daily, morning and night, he punctured a 200 I.U. capsule of vitamin E and rubbed it gently onto the afflicted side of her face. He did not treat the other side. Within several weeks friends began to notice that the woman's skin disturbance was not only improving, but more surprising, the lines on that side of her face were disappearing! Within four months the skin disturbance had completely cleared and all who knew her were exclaiming that there was not a line left on that side of her face. The other side, untreated, was still deeply lined.

This gave me an idea. I called a number of people, telling them the story and asking them if they would be willing to "guinea-pig" the vitamin E skin treatment in the short time we had left. All agreed. The group included several women, two men and myself. After cleansing our skin night and morning, we punctured a 200 I.U. vitamin E capsule with a pin and applied it, morning and before bedtime, to various areas of our faces. Within approximately four weeks, when we could delay the book no longer, I collected the reports from each person.

All who had used the vitamin E twice daily, every day, were enthusiastic. Those who used the vitamin on lines under the eyes said the lines were smoothing out. One woman found that the vitamin tightened her crepey skin. Another reported that it smoothed out the tiny lines on her upper lip. Another woman, who had been sallow, used it all over her face and said her skin was acquiring a rosy glow. She commented that the application of the E made her face feel warm. Still another applied it to her ragged cuticles with excellent results. Some applied their favorite cream or moisturizer over the vitamin E. Others did not.

Those who used this method in a hit-or-miss fashion did not achieve the same results. All others consider it a find of a lifetime.

So it appears that all vitamins, used inside as well as out, have some influence on beautifying skin.

Now let's see how else beauty can be achieved by external methods.

13 Can You Rebuild Your Skin and Hair?

Skin experts once believed that it was impossible to "feed the skin."

To prove that the skin can absorb nutrients, four researchers at Squibb Institute for Medical Research experimented with rats. The rats had been first fed on a diet deficient in vitamins B and D. They were tested, and their bodies, as a result of the deficient diet, were found lacking in these vitamins.

Skin areas were shaved, the missing vitamins were rubbed onto the skin (the rats were prevented from licking them off) and after a period of only two hours the rats were retested. The levels of both vitamins had risen in the body. The only way they could have gained entrance was by penetration through the skin.

During World War II, some prisoners in a concentration camp, subjected to severe malnutrition, lost their ability to assimilate many nutrients by mouth. But when the nutrients were *rubbed on the skin of the inner thighs* of the prisoners, the nutrients were absorbed into their bodies.

As a result of such studies, the Food and Drug Administration now allows vitamins to be added to cosmetics. Other substances can be absorbed by skin and hair, too. I learned this from an experience of my own.

I was lecturing at a convention in Honolulu. A consultant on hair and skin chemistry, Boyd B. Watson, appeared on the same program. He told of new findings about the application of protein to skin and hair which were producing excellent results. He stated two important facts: (1) normal, healthy skin and hair have an acid mantle, and as long as it remains acid, it can help skin and hair maintain health and beauty; (2) chemical analyses reveal that both skin and hair are approximately 98 per cent protein. Protein can be applied directly to the skin and hair, he said, to help them repair themselves. But, he warned, in order for good results, *both protein and acid must be present to work together*. This ties in exactly with what we have been discussing in previous chapters: the need for both protein and acid in the body.

Mr. Watson displayed some skin and hair products containing protein and acid. He spoke to the convention in the morning, which turned out to be fortunate for me. I was scheduled to speak in the evening, and due to the high humidity in Hawaii, my own hair, normally presentable, was limp and bedraggled. After hearing Mr. Watson's lecture, I gathered up his products, rushed to my hotel room and set to work. I used everything from the shampoo to the conditioner and finally the wave set. When my hair was dried and combed, I could not believe my eyes. In one application only, my hair had improved unbelievably. It was glossier, with more body. I appeared proudly on the platform that evening because my hair looked better than it had for years, even though in the nonairconditioned hall the heat and humidity were intense—a combination which would have normally made anyone's hair wilt.

Later, when I returned home, I began trying the protein-acid approach on my skin. It, too, has been improving.

I learned that the products and much of the information presented by Mr. Watson had originated with Jheri Redding, an American chemist noted on the mainland for his discoveries in the field of beauty. In addition to his commercial formulas, available in some beauty salons, Mr. Redding has published formulas which you can make in your own kitchen to beautify your skin and hair. Some of these recipes appeared in an article in a 1964 issue of *Pageant*.

June Wilkie, the author of that article, cited her experience with the Redding formulas. She wrote, "At first I viewed Redding's theories with the same trust I would have placed in the hordes of Genghis Khan. But skepticism began wilting when I watched Mr. Redding drop a strand of hair, which looked like something snipped from an Egyptian mummy, into his conditioner. Before my eyes, the hair turned into a shining example of crowning glory.

"All doubts have since disappeared, for I have tested in my own kitchen the ideas in this article. I have 376 less wrinkles (I was in singularly bad shape) and my hair is now in tasteful condition."

I too, have tested the kitchen-made formulas of Jheri Redding as well as his commercial products. I am just as enthusiastic as June Wilkie.

Jheri Redding, who introduced natural beauty products to beauty salons, has now shifted his attention to providing the public with natural foods and supplements for both health and beauty. Others, including Don Sullivan, a former Redding associate, are carrying on the Redding concept in supplying natural beauty products to the salons.

SOME COSMETICS CAN BE DANGEROUS

Later, I will share with you some of Jheri Redding's formulas. But first I want to sound a solemn warning. Many cosmetics can be harmful. Manufacturers know that most women (even some men) are pushovers for any product which will promise to improve their appearance. Unfortunately, because they know that women will spend any amount of money to acquire beauty, promoters take advantage of this weakness. I am told that one manufacturer has said something like this to his chemist: "If you can come up with a new product which promises women beauty, never mind what's in it, we can sell four million immediately." And they can.

The profit on most cosmetics is fantastic. They often cost little to make and are sold for comparatively staggering prices. A profit of 2,000 per cent is not unusual.

The *Drug and Cosmetic Industry Journal* once stated: "The cosmetic industry has no trouble selling a quarter's worth of toilet water in a one-dollar package for twenty bucks. And the public likes it!"

Senator Maurine Neuberger told the Senate Commerce Committee that, in her opinion, American women were not getting their money's worth for the 2½ billion dollars they spend annually on beauty preparations.

Unfortunately, many cosmetics do not live up to their claims. Still worse, in the manufacturers' haste to make money, the safety element is often ignored. Some products have proved to be downright dangerous.

James Burks, M.D., warns in the *Journal of the Southern Medical Association* of one hazard, ammonium sulphide, which appears in deodorants and other cosmetic products. For some people it may cause itching, swelling, rash, and cracking of skin. Dr. Burks also warns against indelible dyes in lipsticks. These dyes, he says, are photosensitive and cause cracking, drying, and peeling. I personally know two women who used these lipsticks as long as three years ago. Today, their lips are *still* peeling. A man who has learned of these dangers now refuses to kiss his wife unless she wears a natural lipstick.

Other possible dangers, according to Dr. Burks, lurk in some nail polish. It has caused dermatitis not only in the women who apply it, but also in their husbands and children whom they touch!

Another physician, Dr. Paul Lazar, reports in a medical journal the serious reactions in his patients to a commercial nail hardener. A chemical in the nail hardener turned the nails blue and produced such pain that one woman was unable to put on gloves. It took six months of treatment before the allergic symptoms disappeared.

Unfortunately the consumer cannot screen injurious ingredients for himself. To protect trade secrets, labels are usually not required on cosmetics. Natural, safe products are often available only from health-food suppliers.

I, along with others, have been a victim of deleterious cosmetics. In one instance I ran out of my usual brand of natural skin cream while I was traveling. I went to a drugstore and asked for a temporary substitute. The clerk, a woman, handed me a jar, recommending it. The company was well known and nationally advertised. So I bought it. Two hours after applying it, my face swelled up like a pugilist's and the itching became intense. I went to a local skin specialist who gave me emergency treatment, but even after the swelling subsided several days later it left some facial lines I had never had before.

A friend, recently arrived from Germany, has beautiful skin because she has always used only natural cosmetics. But after coming to America she could not resist a tempting magazine advertisement about a new face cream, promising all sorts of miracles. She bought it and applied it, for the first time, just before she went to a party. During the party her face suddenly started to itch and swell until she could no longer stand it. She excused herself, rushed home, and washed off the cream. Because of her damaged appearance she was ashamed to return to the party.

OTHER HAZARDS

Preservatives in cosmetics are responsible for many allergic reactions. Dyes and other ingredients have also caused trouble. As examples, one product, known as PVP, contained in some hair sprays, has been found to cause lung disturbances.* I have seen a picture of a woman who became permanently bald as a result of a do-it-yourself hair coloring manufactured by a prestigious cosmetic company. There is even danger lurking in applying false eyelashes. They look fetching on others but I am afraid to try them since I learned that a professional dancer became permanently blind in both eyes from using a liquid fixative to apply the eyelashes.

Irwin I. Lubowe, in his book, *New Hope for Your Skin*,** lists the names of many toxic chemicals found in cosmetics:

* Linda Clark, *Get Well Naturally* (New York: Pyramid Books, 1968).
** Irwin I. Lubowe, M.D., F.A.C.A., *New Hope for Your Hair* (New York: E. P. Dutton and Company, 1963).

Aluminum salts
Ammoniated mercury
Barium salts
Beta-naphthol
Boric acid
Cresylic compounds
Essential oils
Formaldehyde
Lauryl alcohol sulfates
Mercuric bichloride
Phenolformaldehyde resins
Phthalates
Phenylenediamine compounds
Polyethylene glycols
Propylene glycol
Salicylic acid
Sulfur
Thioglycolate
Zinc salts

Dr. Lubowe lists three rules for safety:

1. Use the minimum number of cosmetic preparations.

2. Select those made by reputable manufacturers or sold by stores of good reputation. These need not be expensive; the larger chains and ten-cent stores carefully check the quality of their merchandise.

3. When you find a preparation you like and can use without reaction, stick to it.

Poisonous substances in cosmetics not only harm the skin; they can affect the entire body.

Betty Morales and John Clark of Organicville, Los Angeles, explain why: "Few think of the skin as a vital organ; yet it is, and the largest one, at that. Its surface area covers about 19 square feet, and it weighs an average of 7 pounds. It varies in thickness from 1/8th to 1/32nd of an inch, and is laced with myriad nerve receptors that transmit the sensations of touch, of pain, and of temperature. It performs these multiple jobs extremely well, despite being roasted in the sun, made leathery by sharp winds, covered with countless powders, potions, rouges, 'pancake' make-up, and certain 'cancer-inciting' lipstick colors.

"Until fairly recently, science viewed the skin as an 'excreting envelope to protect the organism from external invasion,' not recognizing the skin's need to 'breathe,' or its vulnerability to surface intoxicants. Now the skin is recognized as a two-way-passage envelope covering, and blood tests reveal the presence of toxic materials absorbed into the blood stream through the skin."

Agatha Christie, in one of her inimitable mysteries, many of which are based on historical incidents and other facts—not fiction—tells of ancient methods of poisoning a victim in which no one could trace the cause except the poisoner. One of these methods was to add certain substances, such as belladonna or atropine, to creams and rub them into the skin as cosmetics or "healing ointments." The victim "mysteriously" suffered from hallucinations and other serious side effects.

On the other hand, studies show you can influence skin and hair from the inside of the body. If you take an aspirin, 25 per cent of it will appear in the hair within 9 hours and will require 19 days to be completely eliminated. Of 5 million units of penicillin, 1,250,000 will appear in the hair. No studies have been reported of measurement of the appearance of foreign or toxic substances in skin, but we can be assured that they are also present there.

HOW CAN YOU DETERMINE WHICH COSMETICS ARE SAFE?

Dr. Lubowe explains that the acid mantle helps to protect our skin and scalp from bacterial infection. However, he says, we frequently disrupt this acid mantle by using alkaline substances. Many soaps, detergents, and cosmetics are alkaline when they should be acid. Although there is no way to determine what chemicals are contained in cosmetics, there is a method of testing the acidity (called the pH) of any preparation you use on your skin and hair.

Jheri Redding says, "Cosmetics and hair preparations should have an acid pH. To test them, you can buy Nitrazine paper at the drugstore. It is yellow. When you immerse a small strip of paper in a preparation you are considering, if the paper remains yellow, the product is sufficiently acid, therefore acceptable. If it turns gray, blue, or purple, however, it indicates alkalinity in various degrees and may prove harmful."

You can apply this test to lotions, creams, shampoos, wave set and soaps. The Nitrazine test is infallible. Soap is the least likely to pass the acid test.

D. C. Jarvis, M.D., wrote, "Test the moistened surface of a cake of soap with a strip of the Squibb's Nitrazine paper and you will observe that the paper turns a dark blue, indicating that it is very alkaline in reaction. . . . If the cleansing agent you use on your skin is acid, you present the skin with the element that is normal to it, namely acid. When the skin is acid it appears to attract blood to it, whereas when an alkaline solution is applied, such as represented by [the usual type of] soap and water, the skin is apt to be pale and make-up may have to be used to give the appearance of health. . . . A pale skin generally indicates a starving for acid. If you must cleanse with an alkaline substance, you should follow it by an application of apple cider vinegar and water solution, in order to leave the skin normally acid in reaction."

A new invention is a bar of "soap" which is high in protein, contains acid, but includes no soap at all! Yet it sudses and cleanses admirably. It is completely organic, and nontoxic. Whole families, parents and children, are now using this soap with excellent results. One woman told me that except for eye make-up and lipstick it is her only cosmetic; that her skin has become firmer and younger as a result of its use. My mother is so delighted with it, she leaves it on all day as a skin tightener. Since it is high in protein, contains acid, and is held together with a "health food," it contains only safe ingredients. (This "beauty bar" is available in some beauty salons and health stores.)

YOU CAN REBUILD YOUR SKIN AND HAIR

Scientists are beginning to admit that regeneration of skin and hair is possible.

Howard T. Behrman, M.D., and Oscar L. Levin, M.D., in their book, *Your Skin and Its Care*, say, "A peculiar property of skin is its power to renew itself. That is because of the strong tendency to growth of the deeper layer of epithelial cells. The glands and hair follicles also play an important part in this regenerative process."

Jheri Redding adds, "It has long been known by scientists, dermatologists, and biochemists that the skin is composed largely of protein. . . . the balance is made up of lipids, lipoids, phospholipids, lanolin, and lanolin esters. . . . In science it has been conclusively proven by scientists Ciocca, Edwards, and Herd that proteins [and other substances] topically applied to [the surface of] the skin and hair, readily become an integral part of the structure and rebuild either skin or hair and help restore it to a healthful, normal condition."

So it is encouraging to know that both skin and hair can be rebuilt. But we must choose *safe* substances to apply to our skin. The next chapters will tell you what these substances are and how to use them successfully.

14 Which Cosmetics?

As a reporter, dedicated to the task of finding helpful methods of obtaining health and beauty, I have researched every possible book and scientific journal which might yield help. I have also interviewed several outstanding international beauty experts who believe in the comparatively new and safe concept to which this book is devoted. To learn still more about products reported to be helpful, I have served as guinea-pig for many of them myself, or assigned them for testing to friends, both men and women, who tell me the truth. Needless to say, it has been impossible to try them all or name them all. Therefore, I have used as a guideline those cosmetics which illustrate the *principle* of this new approach to beauty. As these newer cosmetics become known, other companies will produce and perhaps even improve on them. But the underlying concept of feeding the cells and the tissues both from within and without is the same. Therefore, the cosmetics I mention are not intended as commercials but simply examples; a means of educating so that you can learn how to select cosmetics for success and safety.

Individual differences play a part in using cosmetics, as well as food. Some work better for one than for another. Also, we all have certain favorites, particularly make-up items, not necessarily put out by the same company. Thus you will have to experiment until you find what is best for you.

When you have chosen them, and coupled them with the

carefully selected diet discussed in Part I, you should have safe, wonderful results.

HOW TO BEGIN TO DEVELOP BEAUTY

Before you begin to make yourself over, beauty-wise, it is important to review certain important principles we have learned:

1. The skin is a two-way street. Substances fed the body can appear in the skin; substances fed the skin can appear in the body, so choose your cosmetics judiciously.
2. The cells of your body, including your face, are constantly trying to rebuild and regenerate themselves. A complete renewal occurs during every seven years. These cells need proper building material to accomplish their regeneration. You can begin at any time. It is never too late for improvement.
3. The skin breathes and is an eliminative organ. The lungs help to cleanse the waste from the body, but the skin assumes a large part of the burden.

   As proof that the skin breathes, there are several reports of people who have covered themselves from head to toe with gold or silver paint for costume balls. They died because their skin was unable to breathe. Beware of using waterproof, cover-all cosmetics on your face. As proof that the skin is constantly eliminating waste matter, witness the ring around the bathtub, or the dirt in the water after you launder your lingerie or nightwear—even when you do it daily. It makes you feel that you *can't* be that dirty! Those who are too lazy to cleanse their skin or remove make-up every night eventually pay the price with large pores, blackheads, and blemishes. Some people who have begun a regular, deep-cleansing program have found that their skin has improved surprisingly by this technique alone. I have seen before-and-after pictures of teenage acne completely cleared by a regular, correct cleansing program. Aida Grey, the beauty consultant, believes that for beauty and health of the skin, it should be cleansed *every eight hours*.

WHAT TO USE FOR BEAUTY

After you have applied the principle of thorough cleansing, you are ready to put your skin on a new diet.

A few beauticians have discovered that certain foods,

rich in vitamins and minerals, can be applied to the skin (as well as fed to the body) with wonderful results in regenerating skin.

For example, two prominent researchers, Dr. Albert Sobel and Dr. Abraham Rosenberg, proved and reported to the American Chemical Society, that vitamins A and D can be absorbed directly into the skin. They learned that when these vitamins were added to face cream and applied directly to the skin they could often be more beneficial in the treatment of skin disorders than when the same vitamins were taken internally. The reason: Though the average intake of food may often contain adequate amounts of both vitamins A and D, some people (particularly those in middle age and later) do not properly absorb vitamins internally, and their skin may be starving for help. For speedier results, the two approaches can work together: one via your face, the other via your diet.

Cosmetics made of foods such as herbs, fruits, vegetables and nuts, rich in vitamins and minerals and raised organically (i.e., without toxic chemical fertilizers or insecticide sprays), are just beginning to be accepted as "skin food."

Dr. Glen J. Sperandie, associate professor of pharmacy at Purdue University, has reported that cosmetics can be, and should be, good enough to eat. He and his colleagues exhibited cosmetics made from natural foods which were not only safe, but even more beneficial than the usual commercial products. These researchers presented exhibits, including an antichapping cream made from tapioca and a complexion lotion made from fresh peaches-and-cream, to the American Medical Association and the American Association for the Advancement of Science.

Two housewives who were bothered by the many allergies resulting from commercial products started collecting beauty formulas from their grandmothers' cookbooks. Some recipes dated as far back as Cleopatra. All were made of insecticide-free fruits, vegetables, and herbs. This search has skyrocketed from a few kitchen formulas to a huge national industry.

Aida Grey, a beautician of Beverly Hills, California, uses edible substances only for her cosmetics. She has become internationally famous and now has salons also in New York and Paris. According to *Vogue,* French-born Aida (pronounced ah-eed-ah) Grey's Beverly Hills salon sees an average of two hundred faces a day; on Saturday, before a big party, the number may reach three or four hundred. Miss Grey's salon is a local landmark in Beverly Hills. Sightseeing buses point it out along with homes of movie stars. Her list of clients is startling. They include (according to newspaper reports as well as her own records) Jacqueline Kennedy, Madame Nhu, Nancy Reagan (wife of California's governor), the Empress of Iran, Elizabeth Taylor, Marlene Dietrich, Irene Dunne, Jane Russell, Nancy Sinatra, Carole Lynley, Jill St. John, Jane Fonda, Betty Grable, and many, many others. Miss Grey was the first person to make up Marilyn Monroe, twenty years ago. Her clients also include men. Two examples are Frank Sinatra and Cary Grant.

Let me tell you how I first learned about Aida Grey. I am possessed of a shameless and insatiable curiosity about health and beauty. I ask everyone with a beautiful skin, whether I know them or not, what is responsible for it. One woman with a flawless complexion told me that she owed her lovely skin to Aida Grey.

After hearing so much about her great success with faces, from other sources, I decided to pay her a visit. I found her a beautiful grandmother who practices what she preaches. As a result, she, too, has a flawless skin. Naturally I asked her how she accomplished all this good for herself and her famous clients.

She explained that she bases all of her work upon, and achieves the good results from, feeding the skin nutritionally rich foods. She believes that no skin is too young or too old to improve. But again, like the body, she believes the skin must have the proper nutrients for its regeneration. Aida Grey also believes that one should change the diet of the face often; that the challenge of variety creates better assimilation.

In her commercial products and her kitchen cosmetics, she uses fruits, vegetables and herbs rich in vitamins as well as minerals to help the skin stay young and healthy.

Her products include a cleanser which contains cherry extract; a mask to stimulate circulation which is a blend of cucumber, peach, carrot, and pineapple essences; another mask, to tighten pores, which is made of raspberry and is followed by a raspberry frappé moisturing cream. For herbs she relies on oregano and mint.

She also uses apple, milk, honey, oatmeal, and almonds. For minerals she includes kelp. She uses sea-salt grains in soap-cream pore cleanser. She adds ginseng to a moisturizer.

Aida Grey has another cleansing trick up her sleeve, which is needed only occasionally. It scales off the dead layers of skin, which, if allowed to remain, clot and dry complexions and prevent skin elimination. This produces a safe, light peeling. After being allowed to dry on the skin, it is rubbed off with a dry cloth, taking dead tissue and waste material with it.

Aida Grey has found that men respond to these natural products as successfully as women. She believes that men age faster than women, and need skin care, too. She says many men use their wives' cosmetics. One night she answered a knock on the door to find a man who said, "My wife and I have separated. She took her pore cleanser with her. Now my skin is breaking out again."

Aida Grey promptly supplied him with his own jar.

I will give you many of her kitchen formulas, which she shared with me for your benefit, in the next chapter.

Another line of cosmetics, made from flowers, nuts, fruits, vegetable oils, and deep-sea plant life, has a long list of delighted followers. These products are designed to blend with air and water. They are designed to help create a beautiful, healthy skin as well as to protect and renew the skin, as nature intended. They are hand-made and include the natural scalp product, used so successfully to regrow hair (mentioned in a later chapter) as well as the prodigious all-in-one cleanser and moisturizer I myself use.

One of the most perplexing problems in choosing cosmetics and make-up is that you have no way of knowing in advance whether they will be the right choices for *you*. Consequently, most women have shelves loaded with odds and ends of left-over purchases which did not live up to their expectations. A unique service has now changed all this. Patricia Allison heads a beauty "sorority," not only provides all-natural products of the highest quality, but, to keep you from acquiring unwanted cosmetics and make-up, gives you the opportunity to try before you buy. The products are available by mail and free samples are supplied, for the price of mailing. Prices are nominal when you do invest in those items which you found satisfactory by first trying them on your own skin.

One of these products, a clear liquid, is a cellular protein, contains herbs, and is a moisturizing agent all in one.

It seems to help the skin repair itself. In fact it has been used on burns with such success that no scars remained. Another product, used for firming the throat area, comes from Switzerland. It is rich in Swiss herbs and lecithin. There are many, many others. This service also has available a special washcloth which stimulates circulation to the skin as well as cleanses. I would not be without it. The first one I wore to shreds over a period of several years. My new one is one of my prized possessions. I have never found these wonderful cloths elsewhere. They were developed because not only this beauty service, but other beauty experts, believe that washing is superior to using tissues or paper towels to remove make-up. Patricia, who has spent a lifetime developing these cosmetics is now fifty-eight and her unretouched pictures show that she looks half her age.

Two cosmetics imported from England are also unusual; one containing the biochemic cell salts and another, bio-stimulants. These products differ from any manufactured in this country.

WHICH LUBRICANTS ARE BEST?

Natural oils can do some remarkable things for the skin. They come from natural sources such as trees, plants, vegetables, seeds, fruits, herbs, nuts, etc. Commercial creams are usually made from a petroleum base such as mineral oil, a by-product of crude oil. Mineral oil is ineffective on the skin. It is not absorbed by the skin, but remains on the surface only. Thus the skin, when treated with cosmetics containing it, appears dry and seems to age more quickly. If, instead, you use natural oils, the skin will feel different because it is being nourished with oils which are compatible and *can* penetrate it.

As I stated earlier, unsaturated vegetable oils, as well as seed and nut oils, are considered helpful. Sesame oil is particularly valuable. Spanish and other European women, noted for their lovely skin, have used it for centuries. Peanut oil is excellent. The Greeks used olive oil. Virgin olive oil is considered more nutritious by many than the deluxe, highly processed varieties. It is available at most grocery stores and you can identify it by the word "virgin" on the label.

The other oils are available at health-food stores.

BEAUTY SECRETS WHICH WORK

A nutritionist who owns several health stores in southern California is a walking example of what nutrition can do for one who uses it inside and out. In addition to taking acidophilus, plenty of desiccated liver, and a whole array of vitamins and minerals, she uses the following beauty secrets herself and shares them with her customers:

1. Every night she uses sesame oil as a cleanser. She opens a large bottle, takes out just enough to last for a week, and places it by her washbowl. The remainder she stores in the refrigerator to avoid rancidity.

2. She flows the oil liberally onto her face and neck, lets it stand a few seconds, then wrings out two washcloths, one after the other, in hot water, to remove both oil and make-up.

3. She next uses a freshener which tests acid by Nitrazine paper. Apple-cider-vinegar-and-water fulfills this requirement.

4. She then uses a night cream which she has "doctored" herself. To a 4-ounce jar of cosmetic cream made of natural vegetable oil she adds the following vitamins: 10 capsules of vitamin A, 50,000 units potency; and 10 capsules of vitamin E, 100 units potency. She pricks each capsule with the tip of a pair of fingernail scissors, squeezes the contents into the cream, and stirs the contents well.

5. After applying this night cream, she does her face exercises.

6. In the morning she simply gives a quick cleansing with the freshener and applies her make-up, made of natural ingredients only.

She also has gorgeous hair. She believes that the protein, liver, and natural oils she eats contribute to its healthy condition.

The night before a shampoo, she massages the same doctored face cream generously into her scalp. She covers her head with a plastic bonnet or shower cap to help the scalp produce heat during the night and absorb the vitamins. Next day she shampoos her hair with a natural shampoo containing egg (this is made in Europe) and follows with a vinegar rinse.

Result: beautiful hair to frame her beautiful skin.

There are many other good products not mentioned here. By using the guidelines presented in this book you may find those you prefer. The important criterion is: Is the health or beauty product *safe?* With your new-found knowledge as a result of reading this book, you are now in a better position to choose wisely and be a more intelligent consumer. Even if every product now known were listed here (I have not purposely meant to bypass any) the list would never be complete. New products are coming out every day. I hope this same information will be an encouragement to manufacturers to make these products really helpful, not just money-makers. It is possible to make a good product as well as an inferior one; one can be sold as well as another. In the last analysis we must raise, not lower, the standards of health and beauty products.

Now, for help with your special beauty problems.

15 What Are Your Beauty Problems?

Nearly everyone has *some* appearance problem to correct. There are two ways of handling these problems; eliminating them or hiding them with make-up. I shall discuss both. First I will give you beauty formulas suggested by expert skin specialists. Finally I will tell you about make-up and how you, like movie, stage, and television stars, as well as international beauties, can have the same help in learning make-up.

Here are the secrets of how to correct your problems. Try the various suggestions until you find which one is most helpful for your skin.

Eleanor Lambert, the international fashion and beauty

columnist, writes "Since meeting Aida Grey, I think twice before I throw away a scrap of food. That apple peel or grape may be just what my skin is starving for. Miss Grey, the satin-skinned cosmetic expert, is a crusader and inventor of what she calls kitchen cosmetics. She thinks the average housewife throws away daily enough fresh foods to keep her complexion young, smooth, and rosy."

Before throwing away an eggshell, rub your finger over the remaining white and apply it to lines under your eyes. Rub lemon skins or cucumber skins on your hands. Smooth the last few drops of the orange rind on your face; it contains vitamin A.

Rub a few drops of oil on your hands after you make salad dressing. Rub a slice of tomato on blackheads.

Natural foods have definite cosmetic values. Flaked or powdered almonds act as an abrasive as well as a stimulant. Honey has long been known as a skin nutrient. And mint has drawing power.

Strawberries have been known for centuries as a mild astringent. Lemon and other citrus juices have also been used as an astringent as well as a bleach. Papaya is a natural enzyme believed in the early days to heal wounds, a fact recently verified at University of California. Avocados supply unsaturated oil, rich in vitamins A, B, C, and D. Many other natural foods can be safely used to help correct specific defects.

Here are suggestions contributed by various beauty experts. (Some are folk remedies, therefore unlabeled.)

KITCHEN COSMETOLOGY

Acne

Make a face pack of bran (the kind you eat) plus baking soda and water. Mix into a paste and apply to the face, leaving it on for 15 minutes. Rinse with apple cider vinegar and water. The proportion: 1 part vinegar, 8 parts water. (Mr. Francis)

Brown Spots

Rub odorless castor oil or apply vitamin E straight on them nightly. (Emily Wilkens)

Blackheads and Blemishes

1. Glands often secrete more oil than the skin can throw off. This remains in the channel of the pore and will harden if not removed in 8 hours. Air hits the oil, it oxidizes, and you have a blackhead or the beginning of a blemish. (Aida Grey)

2. *For impurities:* Heat honey slightly and then spread over the face. Tap the face gently. This produces a pulling power, which draws the blood to the surface and helps to purify the skin surface. Wash gently with warm water, then rinse with cool. One girl from Belgium attributes her beautiful complexion to this honey mask. Used alone or mixed with wheat germ, honey kills germs, draws blemishes to the surface; tightens; tones. (Aida Grey)

3. To loosen and cleanse blackheads, make a paste of oatmeal, honey, and white of an egg. Apply on your skin, massage for 10 minutes, and remove with tepid water. (Aida Grey)

4. Blackheads respond to a mask of oatmeal-and-water paste, or almond-meal and water, or a combination of the two.

One woman who suffered from a blotchy skin for years suddenly found a solution to her problem. When I asked her for her secret she told me that after cleansing, she splashed vinegar-and-water on her face twice a day and allowed it to dry. She added, "I do nothing else. It is so simple."

You can keep a vinegar-and-water mixture in a jar by your washbowl. (The proportion: 1 part apple cider vinegar to 8 parts water).

Eyes

1. Care of the eyes is very important. Eyes should be bathed and lubricated twice daily. Drink rose-hip tea (rich in vitamin C). Dip eye pads in the left-over tea and apply to eyes. If you buy the tea in tea bags, use the bag, still warm, over the closed lid for two or three minutes. (Aida Grey)

2. Another excellent eye lotion is camomile tea (or tea bags) steeped in hot water for 20 minutes, strained, applied in compress form to the eyes for inflammation or congestion (puffiness). Refrigerate and use cold tea twice

a day for refreshing and toning of the skin tissue around the eyes. (Aida Grey)

Raw grated potato may also be used for puffy or swollen eyes. Make a wet compress of four tablespoons of freshly grated potatoes and place on the eye and eye area for 15 minutes. Rinse with cold water. (Christine Valmy, cosmetologist)

3. *Dark circles:* Half a fresh fig over each eye will help erase these dark circles. (Aida Grey)

4. *Bags under eyes:* Brew a cup of strong rose-hip tea. Soak two cotton pads in it and lie down with these over the eyes. They will reduce swelling, refresh and tighten the skin. (Aida Grey)

5. *Lines under eyes:* Soak gauze squares in strong tea made of eyebright (an herb available from health stores or herbal centers). Lie on a slant board. Apply wet gauze to eye area and keep wet for 30 minutes. (Jheri Redding)

For that crepey look under your eyes (or on the throat) odorless castor oil is a wonder worker. (Emily Wilkens)

Freckles

1. Try lemon juice, an oldtime remedy for bleaching. Lemon skins rubbed over the hands will help bleach, and cucumber skins may lighten brown spots. Buttermilk may also help.

2. In the juice of one lemon dissolve as much sugar as it will hold. Apply mixture to each freckle with a camel's hair brush, several times a day. (An old remedy)

Large Pores

1. Mix almond meal with enough water to make a paste. Apply to pores for 20 minutes. Rinse and apply witch hazel.

2. Mix table salt and buttermilk into a paste. Work well into areas where pores tend to be enlarged. Remove with warm water. Repeat several times a week until condition clears.

3. Put 16 ounces of steel-cut oatmeal (available at health stores) into a blender to reduce to powder. Add 8 ounces almond meal, 4 ounces powdered orris root, one ounce powdered castile soap. Moisten one tablespoon of mixture at a time with water to make a paste. Apply gently with fingertips. Rinse with cold water.

For Smoother Skin

1. One woman reports the beauty secret of a friend with a skin envied by all who know her. She has used this beauty secret every day for thirty years: Dry-grind oatmeal. Add a whipped whole egg. Massage into face and let stand for five to ten minutes. Rinse with warm, then cool water. The oatmeal acts as an abrasive, the egg as a protein.

2. One movie star has a skin which is flawless in the glaring sun, even without make-up. Her only beauty formula is one she borrowed from her grandmother. It consists of 2 parts of rose water to one part of glycerine. After cleansing her skin, she applies a few drops all over her face and works it well into her skin.

(Glycerine has long been used as a rejuvenator of dry, wrinkled leather, but used alone it helps some skins, irritates others. The lotion above, however, is reported helpful by all who use it.)

3. *To soothe skin irritations:* Use skim milk at room temperature. Pat on the face and let dry.

4. *For a face peel:* To remove the tired, dead top layer of old skin, use a mask of mashed papaya. Papaya is an enzyme which literally eats all the skin debris. Allow to remain for 20 minutes before removing. Rinse. (Aida Grey)

5. If you want cream for that skin you love to touch as well as look at, here is a brand-new suggestion. At your health store buy a pound of margarine which contains no artificial flavoring, preservative, coloring, or chemical of any kind. Read the labels until you find a brand which contains soybean oil, soy milk, and lecithin as well as vitamins A and D. The soy products provide oil and protein; vitamins A and D are present; the coloring, carotene, is also a form of vitamin A. Best of all, the margarine contains lecithin, from soybeans, which is found in all healthy cells and tissues of the body. It tends to help plump up the cells. The light salting in the margarine probably attracts and holds water, providing a moisturizing effect. Surprisingly, this combination "skin food" does not leave a greasy residue but seems to sink right into the skin, giving it a marvelous, smooth, silky feel. It also makes a good under-eye cream, helping smooth out tiny lines. If these same ingredients were combined into a

commercial cosmetic you would have to pay a fortune for it.

This "cream" leaves a slight sheen, the way a healthy, beautiful skin should look.

Jheri Redding has another formula for smoothing skin: "Make an herb tea by steeping a handful of rosemary in 4 ounces of water for 15 minutes. Strain, cool, add 1 egg white and 1 teaspoon powdered milk to each 2 teaspoons of tea. Mix—don't beat. Store in the refrigerator." Mr. Redding believes that this mixture, used twice weekly, will improve the texture and smoothness within a week.

Sallow Skin

1. Apply buttermilk or milk of magnesia as a mask. Wash off after 20 minutes. (Aida Grey) (Also see oily skin).
2. Apply yogurt and leave on all night. It acts as a bleach.

Skin Discoloration

According to Miss Grey, vitamin B taken internally helps attack skin discoloration. To remedy, she drinks 2 teaspoons of brewers yeast in fruit juice daily, and includes wheat germ, fresh peas, and fish in her diet.

On the face she applies a paste of fresh peas or a pack of wheat germ and honey for stimulation.

To Tighten and Tone Skin

1. Beat together 1 egg, 1 tablespoon milk, 1 teaspoon honey. Apply to face and neck to harden. Leave on as long as you like. Remove with warm water, followed by cold. (This secret dates back to Cleopatra)
2. To plump up tissues, dissolve lecithin granules in warm water, then add to cold-pressed vegetable oil. Rub into skin for all-day or all-night treatment. This treatment needs plenty of time (weeks, months) to help build up the skin.
3. Deborah Rutledge says,* "As far as I am concerned, there is one mask that is the greatest beauty treatment of

* Deborah Rutledge, *Natural Beauty Secrets* (New York: Hawthorn Books, 1966).

them all. . . . My mother has used it for most of her adult life, and I am convinced that is why she has, today, at the age of seventy-six, the complexion of forty, or even younger.

"Doctors are always astounded at the youthful appearance of her skin and truck drivers still whistle at her when she walks down the street. What better testimonial could you want?"

Deborah Rutledge's method of using this is as follows: "All you do is clean your face and smear it with raw egg white. Leave it on for 10 or 15 minutes—or longer if you want to, and then rinse it off with tepid water. . . . After you remove it, your skin is baby soft, looks clean and fresh and smooth, and feels wonderful."

Deborah Rutledge says this mask works wonders if you leave it on all night; used before an important date even even for 10 or 15 minutes, it temporarily smooths out wrinkles and lines.

Skin Tightener

Beat together 1 egg white, 1 teaspoon of spirits of camphor, 1 heaping tablespoon of skim-milk powder, a few drops of mint flavoring. Apply a thin film of odorless castor oil to your skin. Follow with a thick layer of the above mask. Lie on your beauty-angle slant board for 15 minutes. Wash off mask with warm water, followed by witch hazel. (Emily Wilkens)

Oily or Problem Skin

1. Apply a purée of tomatoes or lemon to correct an oily, sallow skin. (Aida Grey)
2. *Wheat germ mask:* 1 tablespoon of wheat germ powder and 1 tablespoon of yogurt. Mix well, apply to the skin for 15 minutes, and remove with tepid water. (Aida Grey)
3. *Lotion formula:* 3 ounces of cucumber juice, 3 ounces of distilled witch hazel, and 1½ ounces of rose water.
4. Three or 4 tablespoons of brewers yeast diluted to make a soft dough. Apply as a mask to face and neck for 20 to 30 minutes. (Diane Rashey)

Dry Skin

1. English women, living in their moist, foggy climate, keep their rose-petal skin longer than those who live in dry climates. The fog also filters out the drying, intense sun rays. If your skin is already dry, use a moisturizer. Arlene Dahl, the movie star-beauty columnist, believes that women should wear a moisturizer 24 hours a day.

2. A vitamin A deficiency can cause dryness. Adding vitamin A to the diet increases sheen in skin and hair.

3. You can also apply directly to the skin by making a mask of fresh or dried apricots (rich in vitamin A) soaked in water for two hours. Mix with honey and apply to the skin as a mask. Leave 20 minutes and rinse off with lukewarm water. (Aida Grey)

4. Use a mashed banana or peach in olive oil and apply as a pack. Let stand for 15 minutes and wash off with lukewarm water. (Aida Grey)

5. Another dry-skin treatment: Use a mixture of milk and melted butter.

6. To the brewers yeast dough (see Oily Skin, No. 4 above) add: olive oil or almond oil plus 1 teaspoon honey, 1 teaspoon lemon juice, mixed with rye flour. Remove with a warm tea made from rosemary leaves. (Diane Rashey)

The following formulas were contributed by Aida Grey:

7. *Dry-skin lines:* Prepare a well-beaten egg yolk with olive oil; apply and leave on your skin for 10 minutes. Follow with a stiffly beaten egg white, spread evenly, and allow to dry for another 15 minutes. Remove with tepid water.

8. *Rough, scaly skin:* Give yourself a mayonnaise facial; massage well into the skin and leave on for 15 minutes. Rinse thoroughly in tepid water.

9. *Dry-skin moisturizer:* Herbs with milk—steep sage in hot water, keep in a cool place for 24 hours, drain, and daily mix a little with sweet cream or butter. Keep the solution refrigerated. Sage is astringent as well as healing. Mint or carnations could be substituted for sage.

10. A good mask for a dry skin is egg yolk and lecithin. Cleopatra used polyunsaturates for her skin—such as sesame oil or olive oil, which she allowed to remain on her skin for 20 minutes and then scraped off with a spatula.

A puree made of 1 banana and 1 papaya, peach, or avocado, applied to the skin and allowed to remain on for 20 minutes, then washed off with tepid water and followed with margarine or any polyunsaturated oil, will relieve the dryness and improve the texture of the skin.

FOR DRY SKIN—MOISTURIZE

Encourage moisture in your skin. Moisturizing has become a household word these days. Yet it is a comparatively recent discovery. The old theory was that lubrication for skin was sufficient. For centuries women slathered oils and creams on their faces without achieving desired results. Then a Harvard dermatologist, Irvin H. Blank, M.D., made a monumental discovery. He took some samples of calloused tissue from the bottom of a foot and immersed it in various kinds of oil. Nothing happened. The callous still remained tough and brittle. Then he dipped another sample of the same calloused tissue in plain water. Soon the callous became soft and flexible!

In the *Journal of the American Medical Association* he writes, "It can easily be shown that neither an externally applied oil or the natural oils can keep the skin flexible without the aid of water. . . . The application of a film of oil to the skin surface relieves the *symptoms* of dryness and the skin seems smoother. The oils may also prevent unwanted water evaporation from the skin."

Dr. Blank states that not all water applied to the skin is absorbed; some evaporates. Nevertheless, a moisturizing cream may be a mixture of oil, water, and an emulsifier to keep the two mixed, plus a few drops of perfume.

One of the most beautiful skins I have seen belongs to a co-owner of "Brownies," a New York City health store. This woman bakes bread daily and cooks vegetables by the steam method for their popular restaurant. When I asked her for the secret of her dewy, pink-and-white complexion, she admitted she did not use cosmetics at all. She said, "I am always poking my head into the hot oven or the steam oven." Undoubtedly this brings circulation to her face and the steam contributes moisture. I think of it every time I open the door to the dishwasher after it has finished its job. I absorb as much steam as possible. This principle is no doubt responsible for the success of the large sale of facial saunas into which you can plunge your face for daily steam treatment.

Leathery Skin

Suntan can wreck your beauty. You may not notice it as first, but just give it time. It gradually dries out the oils and moisture in your skin and leads to leatheriness and lines. Witness any fisherman or anyone who works in the desert who is exposed to the sun, day in, day out. They look weather-beaten.

The dewiest-skinned women are those who live in England or similar climates where the air is moist and the sun is filtered, not direct. After finding that too much sun can cause skin cancer in some, women are waking up. They are wearing hats if long exposed to the sun. Victorian women learned this years ago when they wore big, floppy hats or carried parasols. A few minutes in the sun for vitamin D is enough. Your arms and your legs can pick up what you need without ruining your face.

Vogue magazine says about sun: "It *does* wither skin, with effects so profound that dermatologists describe it as 'premature senility.' Get a swatch of biscuit beige and match your sunning skin to it. Let it get no darker."

A dermatologist, also writing in *Vogue*, says, "Sun worshiping is the single most destructive skin force in this country. I have nothing against a healthy tan, providing it is healthy and not a burn, but I do deplore people playing 'Sun-Dial.' They are headed for trouble, premature aging, skin cancer."

Amy Vanderbilt in her column states that some brown spots, usually called liver spots, are actually "actinic keratoses" or pigmentation caused by overexposure to sun of certain skins, usually very light ones. Such damage can be done at an early age, a dermatologist told Miss Vanderbilt. It may not show up until years later as actinic keratoses. Men are subject to them, also, especially those with fair skins who play golf a lot, sail, or indulge in sports which keep them in the sun.

Chinese women keep their beautiful skin far longer than those of many other nations because they stay out of the sun, or wear hats if they must be exposed to it.

When you are in the sun for an extended time, be sure to have protection of some kind. To prevent leathery skin, one of the best suntan oils is one of the simple vegetable cooking oils. Add a few drops of your favorite perfume.

Hands

Any facial treatment can also benefit the hands. To keep hands young looking, keep them up to prevent bulging veins. (Aida Grey)

Longer Nails and Eyelashes

Norman G. Hillier, author of a book on hair beauty* states, "Hair, skin, nails and all the tissues and muscles of your body are composed of the same substance: protein."

In a New York State University medical study, rats on a low protein diet were found to have slow nail growth. In rats with 8 per cent protein added to their diet, nails grew and were measured. Cold weather and lack of exercise caused nail growth to slow down.

Protein in the form of gelatin has been found helpful, but for safety the gelatin *must* be added to another protein. Gelatin does not contain all the necessary amino acids for body health, hence is an incomplete protein. Growth in rats was severely retarded by feeding them gelatin because of the amino acid imbalance. Milk and bouillon are complete proteins, and when the gelatin is added to either of them all the necessary amino acids are present, producing a complete protein. Protein powders, as mentioned earlier, and mineral supplements have also helped the growth of nails.

One beauty salon, dedicated to the natural approach to beauty, states that apple cider vinegar, applied straight, to the nails, has been known to strengthen them.

Eyelashes can also respond to protein. If the mascara brush is dipped in a protein-rich polypeptide liquid solution, eyelashes are lengthened. This I can also vouch for. It happened to me.

HOW TO REMOVE WRINKLES

There are some skin consultants who claim that once a line appears it is irreversible and can only be camouflaged, not removed.

---

* Norman Hillier, *The Life and Beauty of Your Hair* (New York: Devin-Adair Company, 1957).

One specialist in England writes me, "I do not agree with this concept. The skin is like the cover of a cushion. If the filling becomes loose, the covering will form folds. But if you replace the inner material, you will tighten the outer covering. There are substances capable of setting up intradermal processes which lead to a tightening of the skin due to an increase of subcutaneous supporting tissue."

Wrinkles do not occur overnight, nor can they be removed overnight. With age, plus a poor diet, plus poor circulation, skin can lose moisture and elasticity. Folds and furrows develop as muscles overwork the skin in stress areas where crow's-feet develop from squinting, frown lines from frowning. In youthful skin the elasticity helps the skin to bounce back. In tired, dry, inelastic skin, permanent wrinkles result.

Too much sunlight or lack of moisture can also intensify dryness, compounding the problem. Although the safest way to treat wrinkles is to *prevent* them by breaking facial expression habits and by using correct cosmetics, *they can be reversed,* as you will soon see.

Many wise people start early to use nourishing cosmetics so that wrinkles do not have a chance to develop. A woman in her eighties appeared on television and was asked why she had no wrinkles. She said it was because she had used olive oil on her skin for years.

Lines usually appear in the eye area first because it has no oil glands. Furthermore, according to an eye specialist, there is very little natural circulation to the eye area, including the eye itself.

Protein jellies or creams tend to tighten the skin, according to several laboratories which produce them. Robert Alan Franklyn, M.D., plastic surgeon,[*] states, "If you find there are little wrinkles around your eyes, products with an absorbable base and containing vitamin-rich amino acids (protein) are excellent for smoothing away these skin wrinkles."

Dr. Franklyn contributes a home-made protein formula which he describes as "a marvelous beauty aid which also acts as a facial line eraser." The formula is:

1 egg white
Sweet cream

[*] Robert Alan Franklyn, M.D., with Marcia Borie, *Instant Beauty* (New York: Frederick Fell, 1967).

"Mix the egg white with just enough cream to make the preparation spreadable. Apply to thoroughly clean skin. Let liquid dry on skin for a minimum of twenty minutes, preferably one-half hour. Wash face with tepid water."

You can apply protein, even beaten egg, directly to your skin. There are very few protein creams on the market. One of them, available only from health-food suppliers, is imported from Mexico. It is transparent, contains herbs and minerals as well as protein. Except for a smoothing effect, it is undetectable on the skin, and since so little is needed, a jar lasts indefinitely.

Most exciting is a method for removing wrinkles supplied by Jheri Redding, a chemist, formerly of Redken Laboratories, and author of a forthcoming beauty book: *Botany and Beauty*.

Mr. Redding has proved that protein can help rebuild a protein substance, including skin and hair. Skin takes longer to absorb and rebuild than a single hair shaft, but it does respond similarly in time, he claims.

There are other elements needed by the skin which can be added for faster improvement: unsaturated oils compatible with, and easily assimilated by, the skin; the right proportion of acid (a pH reading of 4.5-5.5) to help absorb protein and maintain skin health; and water, to provide moisture.

Using all of these essentials, Jheri Redding was the first in this country (though later copied by others) to report a skin-building formula, common mayonnaise, which everyone can buy or make for very little money. As proof that it works, Mr. Redding describes a half-face picture of a woman in her eighties which appeared in a European dermatology journal. She had used mayonnaise on half of her face for one year. At the time the picture was taken, the fine lines on the treated side had completely disappeared and the deep wrinkles had become fine lines. The side of her face which had been treated looked as if it were her granddaughter's. The untreated side looked like the grandmother she was.

Jheri Redding tells another story about the use of mayonnaise. He and a companion noticed a waitress with less-than-beautiful skin. Someone had evidently told the waitress that Mr. Redding was a beauty consultant and she asked him to suggest a remedy for her skin. He told her to use common mayonnaise—no other cosmetic.

About a year later, the companion who was with him

the day he made the suggestion called Jheri in great excitement. "Have you seen that waitress you told to use mayonnaise on her face?" he asked.

Jheri answered no; he hadn't seen her since.

"Well, go and see for yourself what has happened."

Jheri went back to the restaurant and almost did not recognize the girl. Her skin looked like peaches-and-cream.

"How did you do it?" Jheri asked her.

"Well," said the girl, "since I work in a restaurant and mayonnaise is always handy, I followed your suggestion and started using it. Every time I had a chance, between customers, I rubbed mayonnaise on my face—often five times a day. I have never spent a penny for any other cosmetic since. And look what happened," she said with shining eyes as she stroked her now-beautiful skin.

WHAT TO USE FOR LINES UNDER THE EYES

Under-eye lines and puffiness are common problems. Jheri Redding says, "Age is one of the prime factors responsible for the lack of 'tone' in your under-eye tissues. If all women, at about the age of 25, would take steps to eliminate the cause, this aging under-eye problem could be vastly improved if not eliminated.

"Cosmetics alone, no matter how perfectly formulated, will not eliminate the problem. Exercise of the under-eye muscles to assist in 'firming up' the tissues in this area is a *must*. Also, a cream formula with an optimum amount of absorbable collagen protein and a penetrating natural oil for restoring the pliability and elasticity of the skin is called for.

"You can make a very effective cream yourself. Start with a good brand of mayonnaise as a base. To the mayonnaise (4 ounces), add 1 ounce of collagen protein. This protein can be purchased from your beauty salon, as it is used extensively by all progressive hairdressers as a treatment for damaged hair, or from health stores. In my considered opinion, it is a must in all of our 'kitchen cosmetics.' It will soon be available in health stores.

"To the mayonnaise and protein combination, add 1 tablespoon of lecithin (liquid type), and blend all of these ingredients thoroughly with a table fork (do not place in blender). Meanwhile, make a strong tea of comfrey leaves or root (4 ounces water, bring to a boil, add 1 handful comfrey leaves, dry or fresh, or 3 tablespoons comfrey root). Both are available from your health-food store. Simmer for 15 minutes. Remove from stove and cool. Add 2 tablespoons of the tea to the mayonnaise mixture and again blend well with a fork.

"Finally, liquefy 1 tablespoon of natural honey by setting a jar containing this amount in warm water. Add to the mixture and stir well.

"The resulting cream-lotion will be an almost perfect application to the under-eye area. It should be refrigerated and should be applied at least twice daily, and once (an absolute must) at night upon retiring. The cream-lotion should be applied generously and massaged into the under-eye area until most of it has been absorbed by the tissue. Don't be alarmed at the slight 'drawing' sensation, this feeling is simply the protein at work. After the first application has been absorbed to a degree, apply another generous amount to the same area to allow a surplus for the tissues to draw on during sleep.

"Now, for another important and very vital part of our regeneration, the exercise of the *orbicularis occuli* (the muscle that encircles the eye). The most effective exercise, in my judgment, is a simple one. Lie down on your slant board for five minutes. Now place the two fingertips of the left hand on the top of the left cheekbone, and pull down with just enough force to pull the bottom eyelid down toward your mouth. Try to close the left eye, but exert enough pressure with the fingertips to prevent the eye from actually closing. Count to six slowly while still attempting to close the eye but prevent it from happening with the pressure of the fingertips. Repeat the same procedure on the right eye with the right fingertips.

"A count of six (if done slowly) is enough. Now apply your 'magic kitchen cream-lotion.' Massage into the under-eye tissue as you do at night and continue to relax on the slant board for an additional ten minutes.

"I have seen this regimen perform what could be likened to a miracle. Just don't expect miraculous results in a few days. It took years for this problem to appear. But do look for unbelievable results in about five weeks.

"In my experience, much more rapid and effective results are obtained if there is an increase of vitamin A intake during your rejuvenation regimen. In fact, a more youthful skin seems to manifest itself if the optimum vitamin A intake is followed throughout life, especially after reaching the age of 25."

Mr. Redding believes that fortified mayonnaise contains *everything* needed for the skin for its regeneration: protein (egg plus the collagenous hydrolized protein in liquid form); unsaturated oil; vinegar for acid; and water. He claims that its daily use will accomplish for nearly everyone the following results:

—Skin will become more velvety within 15 days.
—Elasticity will improve and dryness disappear in 40 to 60 days.
—Definite improvement will be noticeable in 30 days.
—He almost guarantees that lines will be smoothed out and texture will improve in 70 to 80 days.

Mr. Redding warns that deep wrinkles will never be smoothed out completely as long as a person continues to squint, scowl, and grimace—habits which deepen the lines as fast as they are corrected. (One trick to help you break the habit and prevent frown lines from continuing is to apply transparent, magic scotch tape to frown areas during working or sleeping hours.)

Since the wrinkle-removing formula is more effective if circulation to the face is increased, Mr. Redding recommends lying on a slant board for 30 minutes a day, applying the mayonnaise, and ironing out the wrinkles with your fingers.

Sanford Bennett also believed that wrinkles could be rubbed away and that the palms of the hands and the tips of the fingers are the best tools for the purpose. Mr. Bennett recommended the use of a lubricant and tensing the areas to be rubbed to prevent loosening of the skin.*

HOW TO MAKE YOUR OWN SKIN FORMULA

To ensure success of your skin formula, it is important to know what is used in the mayonnaise before you put it on your face. If mineral oil (which is cheaper) is substituted for an unsaturated vegetable oil, it will not work. If some synthetic thickener is used instead of natural egg protein, it will not work. If a vinegar other than apple cider vinegar, which contains some minerals as well as acid, is used, it will provide less nourishment for the skin.

* Linda Clark, *Stay Young Longer* (New York: Pyramid Books, paperback).

So, if you are not *sure* that the mayonnaise of your choice contains these ingredients, there is only one alternative: make your own. It is easy.

Drop a whole egg (fertile if possible, for extra nutrition) into your blender. Add the juice of ½ lemon and a sprinkle of sea salt (also richer in minerals than ordinary salt). Turn on your blender to slow speed. Use whatever vegetable oil you prefer (cold pressed contains more nutrients, including vitamin E). While the motor is still running, pour a continuous, fine stream of oil into the mixture until it becomes very thick. To correct the flavor add some apple cider vinegar, and more salt (also more oil if necessary).

Using this edible mayonnaise as a base, make the following formula for your wrinkle-smoothing face cream:

4 oz. mayonnaise
2 tablespoons of hydrolyzed collagenous protein. (If unavailable from beauty salons or health stores, substitute three more egg yolks.)
2 tablespoons water
A few drops of perfumed oil.
Stir well and keep refrigerated.

You need use this only one hour a day. You may leave it on longer if you wish, or leave it on all night. For best results, precede the use of the formula with a cleansing, using the beauty bar of acidified-protein "soap" also available in health stores. If wrinkles or lines seem to intensify later, it is due to the drawing power of the protein trying to tighten the skin. A temporary booster of a lubricant or water, or both, will tide you over until time for the next application.

One oldtime remedy for wrinkles has apparently been overlooked and forgotten. In our grandmothers' days, women removed stretch marks from their abdomens after childbirth by rubbing cocoa butter into their skin. It is a good lubricant to help restore skin elasticity. It is also an excellent sunburn cream. Never mind if you smell like a chocolate drop. The odor soon fades as the cocoa butter sinks into your skin.

One physician considers cocoanut oil the best wrinkle smoother of all. It is odorless. Both cocoa butter and cocoanut oil are available for pennies at drugstores. Castor oil is also used for this purpose.

LACK OF RIBOFLAVIN CAN CAUSE WRINKLES

Dr. Brady, in his syndicated column, asks, "Why are a few of us at 40 or 50 as wrinkled as dried old prunes?

"In my opinion the most common cause of premature or excessive wrinkles of the face is riboflavin (vitamin B-2) deficiency. Riboflavin is one of the factors of the vitamin-B complex. One rich source of it is milk. One ounce of beef or calf liver contains as much as a whole quart of milk.

"In the early researches on riboflavin, Sherman found that a diet poor in this vitamin produced an 'unhealthy condition of the skin . . . and early development of the physical condition of old age.' McCollum found that riboflavin favored 'preservation of the characteristics of youth.'

"Riboflavin is as essential for the hair and nails as it is for the health of the skin."

WHAT ABOUT HORMONES?

There has been a great deal of publicity about using hormones for youth and beauty. Estrogens, and even progesterone, both female hormones, have been prescribed by some doctors. They have also been added to face creams. I have discussed this with various doctors who are experts on this subject. They are in agreement that around menopause time, the body manufacture of female hormones dwindles or ceases, and the skin reflects this loss.

One physician told me that added hormones definitely can ease a woman through menopause, but, in his opinion, if they are given, they should be *natural*, not synthetic. Another doctor states that no general rules can be made; some women need hormones, others do not; some need more than others. If hormones are given, or in too high dosage, there is threat of cancer in *some* women. Only a physician is qualified to determine these differences and to prescribe and supervise the correct amount if hormones are to be used at all. One hormone specialist told me he objects to large dosages of estrogen, which may not be effective. He finds that a minute dose of any hormonal substance is better assimilated by the body than a large dose, which may be largely rejected. He has had great success with one one-thousandth of the usual pharmaceutical potency. He also feels this small amount is potentially less dangerous.

Skin creams containing estrogen, or both estrogen and progesterone, have been found helpful by many researchers. They believe that if no more than 10,000 units of estrogen are added to the cream, there is no danger. For this reason, this is the highest dosage allowed in cosmetics.

Irwin I. Lubowe, M.D., a dermatologist, says, "It would appear from these findings that various disorders of the skin and hair caused by hormone deficiency could be brought under control by being given the needed hormones artificially; indeed, such procedures have been attempted, sometimes with good effect, sometimes with no discernible result. . . .

"Estrogens taken internally are potent hormones to be taken only under medical supervision. The doctor recognizes that overdosages will throw the entire hormone balance out of kilter, so he will usually prescribe small amounts at first."

Another physician, writing in a medical journal, has stated that hormone creams containing estrogen are safer than taking estrogen internally, and, as far as skin is concerned, do more good.

Robert Alan Franklyn, M.D., plastic surgeon and beauty doctor, writes, "Some women have been happy to find that they have been helped by this auxiliary hormone replacement [via creams]. By now it is pretty well established that this has been done with no untoward results and that repeated use in modest dosage has proved safe.

"Hormones help the skin hold the natural moisture it begins to lose at around age thirty to thirty-five. Generally the effect is to smooth out the skin and erase the lines by 'plumping' up the skin with this vital moisture. The newer hormone creams add progesterone, another potent hormone, to estrogen—which is doubly to the good."*

MAKE-UP

Aida Grey believes that make-up should appear natural, not artificial. She agrees with John Robert Powers, who says that make-up should be called "make-down." In other words, it should be a correction of your faults without calling attention to the make-up itself. Once you know how to correct or camouflage your flaws, as well as find the

* Robert Alan Franklyn, M.D., *The Art of Staying Young* (New York: Frederick Fell, 1964).

colors which match your own present coloring, you should be able to continue the plan indefinitely.

Every season you will see new colors, new make-up fads announced. You need not capitulate unless you wish. Just as in the fashion world, where the length of the hemline and the waistline changes from season to season, so does make-up vary. If hemlines and waistlines remained the same from year to year, women would not have to buy so many new clothes. The clothes industry would suffer economically. The same principle applies to the cosmetics industry.

The world's best-dressed women choose clothes which are becoming to their figures and coloring. They do the same with make-up. Once they have learned what make-up is most flattering to them, they stick to it, unless the skin or hair color changes, necessitating a new plan.

The youngest-looking, most beautiful women I know use a minimum of make-up, if any at all. Joyce Lee, who appears in a later chapter, wears a moisturizer, eye make-up and lipstick, period. Many other beauties do the same. They are proud of the fact that they are bare-faced, wear no powder, and because they are healthy, have no need for rouge. Even Aida Grey, when she finds rouge necessary for her clients, uses such a subdued color, and uses it so subtly, it looks like *you*, not like make-up.

One movie star, well known for many years, still looks young and vital. She says that the older she grows, the less make-up she uses. "Heavy make-up is definitely aging," she states.

Eye make-up can do a lot for a face. Miss Grey suggests using less for daytime, and emphasizing it only for evening, photographs, or professional appearances (television and stage.)

Aida Grey has created a make-up blueprint for members of royalty; society; international beauties; leaders in fashion, business, and the entertainment world. Her unique approach to make-up know-how is now available by mail. Thus anyone, for little expenditure, can be more attractive.

Remember, there are no homely women—only lazy ones.

16 How to Have Beautiful Hair

Hair and skin are mirrors of the condition of your body as well as of your emotions. Stop and think: your hair is a crop that you grow. It draws its growing materials from your blood stream, which nourishes it. But the blood stream itself must contain the proper nourishing elements. If you lack sleep or exercise or follow a poor diet; if you smoke too much or drink too much (alcohol is drying); even if you are perpetually tense, which slows circulation, don't be surprised if your hair looks like a thatched roof.

As one sage has put it, "You can't raise hell and hair, too."

If you add further insult to injury by using chemicals, poisons, dyes, and bleaches, your poor hair does not have a chance.

On the other hand, if you use good sense as well as good products, your hair can be glorious.

Francis Schoenecker, a beauty consultant, believes only in the use of natural by-products of fruits and vegetables. Results are spectacular. Mr. Francis, as he is called, became interested in natural food products for beauty years ago when he noticed that many women had problems with skin and hair and were allergic to various commercial beauty products. To learn more about the subject he took university extension courses in dermatology, anatomy, physiology, and basic chemistry. Later he collaborated in research with a chemist, Stephan Molchan, from southern California, who was also interested in natural beauty products. Together they have reported some impressive results from the use of such beauty aids.

Mr. Francis says,* "People have wondered whether what one eats can help correct hair and skin problems. The an-

---

* Excerpts from Mr. Francis' column in *Pep Talk* magazine.

swer is definitely 'yes.' As in building a house, the material used determines whether the house is of sturdy quality and lovely to look at, or of a shoddy quality and unpleasant appearance. It has often been said, 'You are what you eat,' and to that can be added, 'You are what you think' as well. For emotions can dull the skin, cause rashes and loss of hair and create many other problems in the body.

"Remember, too, that hair and skin problems can be caused by what you *don't* eat as well as what you *do* eat. Good nutrition begins by eliminating the dead foods—white sugar, white flour, empty starches, and all the lifeless over-processed foods which are made from them, including candy and soft drinks. They cause an imbalance in the system and in body chemistry. . . .

"Since the hair is 98 per cent protein, foods high in protein should always be included in the daily diet (meats, eggs, fish, cottage cheese, seeds and nuts). . . . Also, all raw grains, seeds and nuts contain growth factors to furnish hormones, enzymes, vitamins, minerals, many of which are not contained in cooked and processed foods. Because raw nuts, seeds and grains contain iron, silicon, and sulfur, they are considered some of the easiest and safest aids of growing and keeping healthy hair. Raw fruits and vegetables furnish the body with essential trace minerals. Cold-pressed vegetable oils are absolutely essential to the diet. Lack of them causes dull, lifeless hair and parched, rough skin, even eczema. Adding them to salads or even taking them by the teaspoonful has brought dramatic results to skin and hair."

Irwin I. Lubowe, M.D.,* also points out the need of skin and hair for inclusion of all the vitamins, minerals, and protein in the diet; as well as the omission of sugars and starches.

Another beauty operator tells me that when he handles the hair of his customers he can tell what they are eating (or not eating) by the very feel of their hair!

Every hunter and trapper knows that wild animals have poor pelts in seasons when there is a scarcity of suitable food for them.

The first thing a veterinarian observes in a domestic animal is its coat. Is it glossy? If so, the doctor knows the

* Irwin I. Lubowe, M.D., F.A.C.A., *New Hope for Your Hair* (New York: E. P. Dutton & Co., 1960).

animal is in good health. If, on the other hand, the coat or fur is dull, without sheen, then this is a sign that something is wrong with the animal's health. In such an event the veterinarian does not prescribe drugs, he changes the diet. People should be treated in the same way.

W. A. Krehl, M.D., says, "From primitive times, man has related the gloss and sheen of the hair coat and skin of his pets and herds with good dietary practices and good general health. In experimental nutrition studies, a change in the hair coat and skin of animals has often been the first and most outstanding feature of deficiency disease. . . . Because these skin changes have appeared with poor diet, dermatologists have naturally been much influenced by the use of special diets, vitamins and minerals in nearly every conceivable dosage level and combination in an attempt to manage and treat skin diseases."

One company has manufactured a protein powder for dogs. Good results soon become noticeable. The dogs' eyes become more alert, energy increases, and the coats become glossy, thick, and beautiful. Impressed with the effect on animals, the company has now combined almost the same ingredients into a protein powder for humans. The same results occur in people!

WHAT CAUSES FALLING HAIR?

Donald F. Norfolk, D.O., says, "A healthy head of hair is often proclaimed 'Man's Crowning Glory.' But today, though we pour a vast sum of money on our heads in the form of creams, lotions, 'restorers,' dyes and medicated shampoos, it seems to have lost much of its former glory. Man is becoming increasingly bald, while hair which was once soft and sleek is now all too often lank, limp and lustreless.

"The reason is not hard to find. The hair is an extension of the skin. Although largely composed of dead, closely packed cells, these organs are, in fact, alive. They develop from beds of highly active cells, they grow, they wither, and then are replaced by entirely new cells. Yet a large percentage of our modern treatment of the hair is based on the mistaken assumption that the hair is dead. It is not; it is very much alive as long as the body is alive.

"Hair does go through regular, but intermittent cycles

of dormancy, however. After a period of about two years the hair arrives at the end of its normal span of life. The root of the hair dies and becomes detached from the floor of the follicle. As soon as this happens a new hair starts to grow, pushing the old hair in front of it as it develops. Eventually, probably during the act of brushing or combing the hair, the old hairs are shed at a rate of something like forty to eighty hairs a day.

"In health, the rate of growth of new hair balances the rate of hair fall-out, but in sickness [or malnutrition] the falling may become excessive or the rate of regeneration insufficient. Then signs of excessive hair loss and baldness occur. In general, to reverse this condition it is necessary to improve the general health and stimulate circulation to the scalp."

Many women, as well as men, are complaining about falling hair these days. Some cases of hair loss may be a direct result of radioactive fall-out. Dr. Lubowe describes tests with humans and animals who have been afflicted with falling hair or patch baldness following nuclear explosions; eating radioactive contaminated food; or swallowing radioactive iodine as a medical treatment. There is only one known solution to this problem: fortify the body with nutrition so that it can protect itself against the ravages of radioactive fall-out, now a worldwide menace.

In my book, *Get Well Naturally,* I have listed the foods, as tested by scientific studies, which provide this protection. Kelp added to the diet has been found by medical researchers to act as a special antagonist to radioactivity. Protein and vitamins, particularly vitamin-B complex, and brewers yeast, have produced dramatic protection of animals against radiation.

NUTRITIONAL HELP FOR HAIR

Katherine Pugh is a former Powers Model and director of a charm and modeling school specializing in grooming for men. She has written two books* with the sole purpose of helping people grow hair through diet. She cautions that there is no magic pill, nor a single magic food which will do the trick. Even her well-rounded program, which

* Katie Pugh, *Hair Through Diet,* and *Baldness: Is It Necessary?* Available from Mailing Services, Inc., 1524 Brook Road, Richmond, Virginia.

has brought results to many, does not bring overnight success. She feels that hair growth depends on healthy glands. Improving them takes time and patience. She warns that you may not see results even in six months, but by following a health-building diet of protein, and more protein, plus certain vitamins and minerals, hair growth is possible, provided the glands are not already too degenerated or too diseased, and have not been removed by surgery.

Mrs. Pugh cites several reasons for baldness: heredity, lack of vitamin-B complex, dandruff, and multiple nutritional deficiencies. She points an accusing finger at over-processed foods. The secret of growing hair, she says, seems to lie in protein and B complex, along with copper, zinc, and other elements found in natural foods. The two most important vitamins she considers helpful are inositol and choline, but she warns readers not to rush out and buy them and start taking them singly. Eating them in foods containing the entire family of B vitamins is a more reliable method, she believes.

She also cautions against carbohydrates, processed foods, soft drinks, too much coffee, and too many cigarettes. She advocates a diet including the following foods: protein and protein powder, raw wheat germ, brewers yeast, desiccated liver, sunflower seeds or meal, lecithin, kelp, carrot juice, vegetable oils, natural vitamins and minerals, fish-liver oil for vitamin A, and honey used exclusively for sweetening.

One important food substance is cold-pressed vegetable oil. Studies with animals show that if they have been deprived of natural oils which contain linolenic and linoleic acids (better known as unsaturated fatty acids) the hair falls out in patches. But when the natural oils are restored to the diet, hair grows in again and becomes glossy. Cold-pressed oils are available in health-food stores.

There is scientific proof that a person's hair roots reflect the amount of protein in his body. Three nutritional scientists produced this proof at the University of California at Berkeley. They fed one group of men a liquid formula providing 75 grams of protein daily. The control group were deprived of protein. After 15 days, 100 hairs were plucked from each man's head and the root bulb and root sheath examined under a microscope. A higher level of protein was observed in the protein-fed men, whereas in those deprived of protein there was less hair color and the root bulbs were atrophied. This experiment was reported in *Science*, July 28, 1967.

One company has formulated a protein powder combining several forms of vegetable proteins. They call this a "live protein" product because it is not subjected to processing or heat and must be refrigerated. By stirring one or more tablespoons of this protein powder into juice or water daily, and drinking it, some people have told me that their hair stops falling; in other cases thinned-out spots begin growing in again, and the lustre and body of the hair is improved. Best of all, their energy increases.

The powder contains carefully formulated amounts of rice polishings, brewers yeast, wheat germ, dulse (a form of kelp) and finely ground fenugreek, sunflower, and chia seeds.

Although this food may not help everyone, it has been beneficial:

CASE HISTORIES

1. "I am sixty-six years of age and have been 75 per cent bald for the last eighteen years. . . . I decided to try the protein powder. Have been taking it for eight months now. Hair has grown to 3½ inches thick with plenty of long hair and fuzz that has broken through a tight, shiny, bald head."

2. "I will be willing to show anyone the inch or so of hair on a formerly bald head. Certainly as important is the exceptional strength and stamina I now have."

3. "After spending hundreds of dollars at several of the leading hair salons . . . I gave up hope of saving my hair or growing any back. . . . Several months ago I began using this protein powder. It wasn't long before I began to see an improvement both in my hair and in my general health . . . the two bald spots at the back of my head are almost completely filled in. My hair is much thicker . . . more body, life, and lustre. Slowly but surely hair is regrowing in the front where it had started to recede. The powder also gives me loads of pep and energy."

4. "I have been using a protein powder for approximately six months. My hair has lengthened considerably . . . is thicker, looks healthier and is softer. . . . I had tried dozens of different so-called hair restorers during the past twenty-five years, none of them worked. I am better satisfied with the results I am experiencing with this protein powder than any other product I have ever used."

5. "Since using this protein powder I have regrown a

considerable amount of hair on my head, which was quite bald. I am very pleased with the results. I have also had a tremendous improvement in my nails."

Mr. Francis sums up the many causes of baldness: "Statistics show that in America today, there are over 3 million women who are bald, and over 4 million well on their way toward baldness. Some of the chief causes of baldness and damaged hair are:

1. Too vigorous brushing with harsh nylon bristles.
2. Too much sun.
3. Infections and other diseases, high fevers.
4. Lack of scalp exercise.
5. Emotional tensions.
6. Allergies to certain hair preparations such as dyes, hair sprays, etc.
7. Drugs.
8. Continual shampooing with alkalin soaps which remove the protective natural acid mantle; detergent shampoos that strip the oil glands under the scalp; dandruff-removing shampoos that can remove the hair.
9. Harsh chemicals in permanents, bleaches, tints, and rinses.
10. Poor nutrition.

He adds, "My associate, Stephan Molchan, an eminent chemist, has also discovered that even nuclear explosions and fall-out have produced unusual effects upon the actions of some permanents and tints. They color more readily or 'burn.' Some hair products rely on molecular reconstruction and therefore are directly affected."

SAFE TREATMENTS FOR FALLING HAIR

Mr. Francis says, "Occasionally, a client will rush into the salon exclaiming, 'My hair is just falling out by the handful! What should I do?'"

He answers, "If the hair can be pulled out in 'swatches,' without pain, or if the hair is extremely sparse, collecting readily in a bunch, the recommendation would be an immediate appointment with an eminent dermatologist or a family doctor, as the problem could be caused by thyroid malfunctioning, extreme nerve condition, etc.

"If damage is due to tight scalp, which strangles and

starves the hair bulb, heavy dandruff and cradle cap or similar conditions, treatment is within the jurisdiction of the skilled beautician.

"These situations cause inflammation, infection, itching, rash, and unsightly 'salty' shoulders (dandruff). One basic cause is inferior shampoos and improper shampooing.

"Remember dandruff basically is a *normal* skin function, not a disease. It is the sloughing off of matured epithelial cells and food waste products. This is why shampooing is important. A first shampooing removes the lifted waste. The second shampooing removes scalp residue from the first, and leaves a welcome antiseptic action on the infected follicles.

"If hair is not rapidly falling, use a hairbrush to help loosen waste from scalp. Shampoo every two weeks or once a week according to accumulation.

"No detergent shampoos please! Let us help you keep that natural hair on your head, not in your hand."

Mr. Francis continues, "Detergent shampoos turned out to be the villain in the case of three ladies who complained of thinning hair. In the case of two of the women, we discovered they had been using a detergent shampoo for years without knowing it. The third was using a dandruff-removing shampoo. Result—loss of hair. Dandruff-remover shampoos will also remove hair with prolonged use, because of powerful disinfectant or antiseptic action. A good shampoo is sufficiently antiseptic except for unusual instances such as infected follicles and pores.

"Detergent shampoos are harmful to the life of the hair and skin. They strip the oil glands in the scalp of their precious lubricating oils. The American people, even in their overwhelming desire for cleanliness, wouldn't consider buying and using a box of detergent for their faces—why then on the skin of the head?

"If you are a detergent-shampoo user, I suggest that you switch to any of the fine herbal shampoos available through your local health store or health salon.

"If you can't find, or don't have access to the herbal shampoos, then a good vegetable oil shampoo will serve. Or perhaps you are a believer in 'good old-fashioned castile shampoo.' In either case, do what grandma did after shampooing. Use a rinse made of 1 quart of warm water, and 1 tablespoon of vinegar or lemon juice. Remember, the skin and scalp must maintain a 2 per cent acid balance.

"Men frequently ask, 'Doesn't it look like I'm getting bald at the hairline?'

"Research reveals that a man's hairline recedes about one inch at the age of thirty and, with proper care, tends to remain there. In women, this same procedure is postponed until about the age of fifty. So unless there is consistent loss of hair showing on brush, pillow or comb, there is no real cause for alarm. However, if you are losing more than 25 hairs a day with the tiny bulb ends attached, it's time for action. In our salons we use the stimulating natural scalp stimulant treatment. It works wonders."

A RELIABLE HAIR GROWER

The action of this natural scalp stimulant, which contains all natural ingredients, when applied to the scalp, causes the skin to "relax" and the pores to dilate, relieving impaction of roots. A deep cleansing action then removes sebaceous "gum" and the conditioning element helps to control hair breakage. Along with these treatments we recommend that the patron ask a doctor or health store for a good vitamin-mineral capsule which includes copper, iron, manganese, and silicon.*

THE EFFECT OF THE SCALP STIMULANT

Case Histories from Mr. Francis:

1. The hair of one woman was extremely sparse on top of the crown. After a three-month treatment fuzz began to appear between the falling hairs. Soon the hair began to stop falling. One year and two bottles of scalp stimulant later (including use of an all-organic hair color) the hair became luxuriant, far exceeding expectations.

2. A man, age forty, had been bald since high school. Cause: extreme fragilitis. Hair broke off as fast as it protruded from scalp. In just six weeks of using the scalp stimulant, his scalp was entirely covered with fine hair about one inch long. It doesn't seem to get much longer at present, but he is proud of it.

3. An officer of the U.S.N., had been bald for twelve years. . . . no hair on top. Cause: Tight scalp; also apparently undernourished in trace minerals. In addition, he

---

* Mr. Francis sells no products. He is a consultant only.

had always used bar soap for shampoo. He noticed new hair growth in a mere three weeks' use of scalp stimulant and his hair has continued to grow promisingly.

Mr. Francis says failures to grow hair by this method may exist, but he has never known one.

"To us a sincere testimonial is a normal, healthy, and enthusiastic response of an individual who knows the truth from the most reliable source of all—his own experience. In our turn we share these experiences with others as they, too, learn that they can have beauty without the sacrifice of health.

"Through the past four years, it has been a great personal satisfaction to observe the increased hair growth in clients who previously had abnormally thin hair or balding heads. This includes my own wife, who now has more hair than she has had for the past five years—enough to have a pixie haircut. This improvement is just from the use of natural tints and permanents only.

"Those who have used the good, poison-free cosmetic and grooming aids know they must also improve their over-all health. Health and beauty belong together. Results speak for themselves. And satisfied users testify to the facts."

WHAT CAUSES SCALP SUFFOCATION?

According to Mr. Francis, "Thinning spots on the scalp and eventual baldness can be caused by suffocation of the scalp. There are various causes for scalp suffocation. Not always are they easy to recognize by the one afflicted with the problem.

"We have found in making a hair analysis of customers suddenly concerned with obvious thin spots, that the scalp area had been completely impacted and sealed. In particular cases this was due to certain color rinses being applied to the hair. Residue of the rinse still covered the scalp.

"Not all rinses cause this type of problem, of course, but where it happens, the rinse coats the scalp with a very fine plasticlike film, almost totally sealing off the activity of the scalp. Then, if the hair is washed only about once every two weeks, and the scalp not thoroughly scrubbed of the rinse during the shampoos before the next rinse is applied, a state of impaction builds up that causes the scalp to become hard and sore as well as choking the hair roots. If the circulation to the roots is completely cut off, the roots die, creating a bald spot.

"A recent patron had this particular problem due mostly to the fact that she was extremely hesitant about scrubbing her scalp, when she found that thorough scrubbing lightened the color of the hair rinse previously applied. Not realizing the danger involved in the lack of thorough scrubbing and sincerely desiring to maintain a consistent hair color caused her to end up with large thin spots.

"To correct the problem, we advised a heat cap and hot cleansing material for twenty minutes. This relieved the tightness and started the proper functioning of the oil and sweat glands, thus lifting off the impacted scalp covering.

"A later examination of the scalp revealed minute hair filling in the balding spots. The scalp was also in a much more relaxed state.

"Since the patron did not wish to continue without a hair tint, we advised a 'soap-cap' which consisted of a nonallergic tint, mixed with an herbal shampoo. This gave a satisfactory tint.

"A good rule to follow is the one cooperating with the natural laws of the body. Keep the scalp free of impaction through proper shampooing and brushing. Treat your scalp well, and it will treat you well.

SOME REMEDIES FOR FALLING HAIR

Jheri Redding has a treatment which he claims is equivalent to seven hours of daily stimulation, and will stop falling hair in 87 per cent of the cases. He admits that it will not reverse baldness if hereditary.

Here is his formula: "Mix 4 ounces of red cayenne pepper with a pint of 100 proof vodka. Every day for two weeks, shake the mixture several times, then strain, preferably through a nylon stocking until the liquid is free of pepper. You now have liquid capsicum, and cheaper than it would cost to buy. (Don't drink it.) Each morning and evening apply the mixture to the scalp areas threatened with baldness. Within five or six weeks, there should be new hair."

Another natural remedy for falling hair was contributed by Mary Haworth in her newspaper column. It is a combination of white iodine and castor oil. She writes, "Every other day for five days apply white iodine to the scalp with a swab of cotton. Part the hair in small sections to be sure that the iodine reaches the scalp. On alternate days apply heated castor oil in the same way.

"On the fifth day, massage the scalp liberally with more castor oil and follow with a hot towel treatment or put on a plastic shower cap for a minimum of an hour—longer if possible—to bring the heat to the scalp. Then shampoo the hair.

"The white iodine stops the hair from falling. The castor oil plus heat stimulates new hair growth. In any case [she says] the iodine seemed to stop the hair loss almost at once, but it is too early yet to measure the growth of the new hair."

WHAT ABOUT WIGS?

One physician has noted that wearing tight hats which bind the head, by slowing down or cutting off circulation to the scalp, is a sure method of producing baldness. Wigs are more binding than hats, and worn for longer periods. It is true that though wigs can be a convenience, many women are reaching the point where they dare not appear in public without one, because often their hair is ruined, stiff as straw and ugly as sin. When human hair is bought to make wigs, the hair of American women cannot be used. Only hair grown by European women, who still treat it naturally, and live on a good diet (a tremendous influence on the condition of hair) is considered sufficiently beautiful for wig-making.

The trouble is that demand for beautiful hair is beginning to exceed the supply. The hair of young girls in Spain is particularly desirable. Not only does bargaining take place with the mothers for their daughters' hair, but, this failing, "hair raiders" have actually held up girls at night and chopped off their hair. The hair is sold to wigmakers for very high prices with no questions asked.

Jheri Redding believes that there is decided danger in wearing wigs. The hair breathes, but wigs prevent it from breathing. The solution, he says, *is not to need a wig in the first place,* except as an occasional cosmetic change.

Women should, and can, have such beautiful hair they should be proud not to wear a wig! The following pages show you how.

17 How to Recondition Hair

Mr. Francis advises, "To recondition hair, one must not only understand how best to correct the unwanted situation, but the reasons why the hair became problem hair in the first place. Much is heard over television about beauty aids that produce lovely hair. However, beauty aids should be as carefully chosen as your health-giving foods. If not, they can be a contributing factor, or even the factor itself, in creating problem hair."

Do not believe everything you read or hear in commercials about hair (or skin products). Many manufacturers find it difficult to judge the merit of a product objectively when their livelihood depends on its sale. Nature is safer.

"When the hair is 'dry' and 'lifeless,' it is often due to poor cleansing agents—the result of lack of knowledge in selecting the proper beautifying products. Men, too, have this problem, as they are prone to use alkaline bar soaps on their hair.

"Dry hair basically is the lack of moisture, protein, and natural oils. Too-frequent shampooing contributes to that rough, dry feeling, especially if detergent-type shampoos are used. They strip the fatty oil glands under the scalp.

"To shampoo hair properly, lather with a 'non-chemical' shampoo, two or three times. Let the last lathering soak a few minutes to help 'lift' the dead skin cells. Then rinse thoroughly.

"To cleanse the scalp between shampoos, thoroughly brush the hair each day. This removes dead skin (normal shedding) and spreads any excess scalp oil evenly, relieving dryness. The circulating blood brought to the scalp by brushing will also nourish the hair.

"Lack of scalp oil due to 'plugged' or covered oil glands is another factor that causes dry hair. If such is the case, a scalp treatment is in order. To remedy this particular condition, we use natural pore-cleansing agents along with a heat cap for a dilating and perspiring effect. Some salons do this.

"Should the problem be that of damaged hair, avoid using 'grease,' 'hair oil,' etc. You need the use of a protein conditioner to return what is lacking in the hair. These conditioners are available at local health stores and natural beauty salons. For damaged hair due to overbleaching, tint, or waves, a special salon recovery treatment consisting of protein is given.

"However, while hair problems can be corrected, prevention is still the best method to follow. Learn the natural laws of health, follow them, and your hair will always be in good condition."

To save beautiful hair, you can take these steps:

Step one: Watch your diet. Choose the correct foods recommended by hair authorities.

Step two: Be sure your scalp is sufficiently acid. How do you know if your scalp or hair is acid? D. C. Jarvis, M.D., answers, "The skin which is alkaline in reaction will itch. An itching of your head or skin surface of your body is the body's way of announcing its lack of acidity. Apple-cider-vinegar-and-water solution will stop it."

Always use a vinegar-and-water rinse. If you are a blonde, lemon juice in water may be substituted.

Step three: Use a shampoo which tests acid with Nitrazine paper.

Step four: For reconditioning hair, particularly if it is dry, use an ordinary mayonnaise, purchased at a grocery store. It contains many helpful ingredients: egg (protein), vinegar (acid) and vegetable oil.

Jheri Redding suggests this procedure: Shampoo and towel dry your hair. Apply the mayonnaise—plus a tablespoon of collagenous hydrolyzed protein (polypeptides) and leave on ½ to 1 hour. Then shampoo lightly and rinse with an apple cider vinegar rinse.

OTHER HAIR PROBLEMS

Here is help from Redding for other hair worries: If your hair is too oily, dissolve a tablespoon of salt in the skim milk used as a wave-set.

According to Redding, your hair has a salt bond and a sugar bond. If your permanent takes the life out of your hair, it may be because you need to re-establish the sugar bond. This is done by applying blackstrap molasses to your hair. Let it stand for an hour before rinsing with vinegar water.

One beauty operator wrote him: "When I first read that blackstrap molasses could help strengthen and re-establish the sugar bond or restore the condition of hair damaged by a permanent, I decided this was *too* much to believe. You can imagine my surprise when I tried it on my own hair, which was in terrible condition. It worked! I have used it since, many, many times, and it is like magic."

Jheri Redding's conditioning formula for dry scalp and very brittle hair is:

½ ounce apple cider vinegar
½ ounce glycerine (available from drugstore)
 3 ounces of polypeptides (available from some beauty
    salons and health stores)
½ ounce corn or wheat germ oil

First shampoo hair with acid-balanced protein shampoo. After the second soaping, towel dry and apply above formula. Leave on hair at least 20 minutes so that it can penetrate the hair shaft. Rinse and set.

WATCH THOSE COMMERCIALS!

Choose your hair products with great care.

Dr. H. I. Silverman, Professor of the Research Institute at Brooklyn College, reports research information about the effects of commonly used hairdressing ingredients. His studies show that:

—Liquid lanolin increases the hair strength by 2.4 per cent.
—Olive oil increases hair strength by 1.9 per cent.
—Castor oil increases hair strength by 9.2 per cent.
—Mineral oil does nothing; it neither increases nor decreases hair strength.
—Alcohol decreases hair strength by 9.1 per cent.
—Water decreases strength of hair by 7.7 per cent.

This last finding (i.e., that water decreases the strength of hair) would suggest that hair should not be shampooed oftener than necessary. Cornell University supports this by a study which showed that in each shampoo with soap or the average commercial shampoo the following nutrients were lost from the hair and recovered in the shampoo water: calcium, phosphorus, iron, and nitrogen.*

MY EXPERIENCE

The hair treatment which revived my hair so magically while I was in Hawaii was this: I used a protein-acid shampoo (it comes in a concentrate to which you add water), plus 4 drops of avocado oil. After a second soaping I stripped my hair of suds and applied two tablespoons of collagenous hydrolyzed protein liquid to my hair and left it ½ hour. I then used a vinegar rinse and set my hair with the protein wave-set.

If you cannot find such products in a beauty salon, either ask the salon to order them or substitute kitchen remedies.

Instead of the liquid protein beat three raw eggs and massage into your hair, leaving for the same length of time (½ hour or more), so the protein can penetrate the hair shaft.

If you cannot find an acid-base-protein shampoo, shave castile soap and dissolve in water (don't use directly from the bar; it will dull hair). Use apple cider vinegar in the rinse water.

For a wave-set or to give body to the hair, there are several possibilities.

HOW TO GIVE BODY TO THE HAIR

Mr. Francis recommends making your own wave-set. He says, "Flaxseed obtained from your local health food store makes the perfect wave-set. This is used in many natural salons: A cup of the flax, either ground or whole, added to 3 cups of water and boiled, may then be diluted to the desired consistency with water. Egg white also works, but leaves the hair with a little 'heaviness' when dry. Smooth, plastic rollers, instead of the brush rollers, will eliminate fuzziness, if that's a problem. However, a set will last longer with brush rollers."

To add body to your hair you can either use the protein wave-set jelly or protein hair spray. Or, Jheri Redding suggests using skim milk as a wave set. Don't rinse it out;

* Linda Clark, *Stay Young Longer* (New York: Pyramid Books, 1968).

allow it to dry. If this doesn't provide enough body, or doesn't last long enough, he suggests getting still more protein into the hair by making a paste of dried skim milk powder and water and applying it to your hair as a pack for 20 minutes. If this fails, there is still a stronger formula: Redding suggests an application of wheat germ oil, rinsed out with vinegar solution.

Still another kitchen formula for setting hair: *Vogue* has reported that one prestigious beauty salon in New York City gives its clients a choice of colors and flavors of wave-set which they apply to the patron's hair in the salon. According to this report, the "set" is Jello. Since the base is gelatin, it contains protein. Lemon or lime should also contain acid. If the hair is damaged by a permanent, the sugar should help correct this condition, as we have already mentioned. This type of wave-set is, according to *Vogue,* also quick-drying.

Mr. Francis summarizes the essentials of reconditioning hair, in order to make it beautiful and keep it beautiful.

"To help ensure a healthy, shining head of hair, regardless of your age:

1. Brush daily and massage. Brushing is one of the million-dollar secrets toward beautiful hair. Brushing squeezes the oil glands in the skin, carrying the precious oil to the ends of the hair, conditioning and cleansing it. Be sure to use a natural-bristle brush. Healthy hair stands out naturally from the head rather than lying plastered against the scalp.
2. Shampoo once a week or every two weeks using natural herbal shampoos. If not available, use castile followed by lemon or vinegar water rinse.
3. Use only natural permanents, tints and hair aids.
4. For severe baldness, consult a dermatologist.
5. Where needed, have hairdresser use the natural pore cleansing and protein treatments, and the "heat cap."
6. Use proper nutrition and supplements.

"Hair beauty and good health go hand in hand. One complements the other."

Now that you are on the road to acquiring beautiful texture and gloss, natural coloring and permanents are safe as well as successful.

18 Safe, Beautiful Permanents and Hair Color

Because I consider Mr. Francis' approach to beautiful hair safe, I asked him questions which I felt were of vital interest to everyone. Here are my questions, and his answers:

Question: Are all permanents safe?

Answer: No. A statement from the *American Medical Association Journal* discussing thioglycolic acid (a substance in chemical permanents) points up the necessity for healthful beauty products.

Now that this product (in home permanents) is being sold in the chain stores, its indiscriminate use will result in an increased incidence of poisonings, many of which are already finding their way to the courts. Adequate labeling and understanding of the dangers involved are imperative. The process has been applied to many thousands without ill effects, but it seems probable that repeated exposures may eventually prove disastrous to those who have been immune up to the present time. Those with anemias and allergic disturbances were the most vulnerable.

Also in the *American Medical Association Journal*'s report were case histories of people suffering with thioglycolic acid poisoning following permanents. One case suffered from loss of hair, cramps, lymph disorder, and scalp itch. Another developed a violent blood imbalance, and at time of the *Journal*'s writing had shown no improvement.

It is my firm conviction that *safe*, scientific beauty aids should be available everywhere. There is no longer any reason to sacrifice health in order to obtain beauty.

Occasionally we see fine hair partly or totally devoid of inside "core" sections, due to the physical make-up of the individual. Even a good operator may overprocess this type of hair, waiting for a good test curl.

When the solution is on, the layers of protein cells are disconnected from each other, and must be firmly reattached with the neutralizer to a good base such as the outside of the hair as well as the core. Some hair may possibly not have a core. If this is the case, then an osmatic permanent would work best as it uses no thioglycolic acid to further injure hair.

I use a special permanent which does not contain thioglycolic acid. It does not require the operator to wear rubber gloves. It does not kink, frizz, or break the hair. This type of permanent does stop existing breakage and prevents further breakage. It contains no acid used in the cold waves, and requires no heat of the machine wave. It is absolutely nontoxic.

Question: Is bleaching harmful?

Answer: Yes. The chemical bleaches burn out good protein cells that are difficult to replace. This may not at first be obvious, but soon is felt in dryness of hair and loss of elasticity. Where there is continual bleaching and overlap of already bleached areas, severe hair breakage results. Hair becomes hollow, loses its natural sheen, and the beauty operator must try to fill in the "burned-out" cells in order to ensure a good take in bleach and curl.

However, there is no need for this crime against hair. Vegetable bleaches made from pure vegetable materials such as alfalfa, tomatoes, etc., are now available. They contain no harsh acids, chemicals, or peroxides.

Hair bleach often causes trouble. In some people it can cause a rash of small, uncomfortable, and unsightly blisters. In particularly sensitive people these disturbances sometimes appear even before the bleach job is completed.

Bleached hair cannot always be permanent-waved, particularly if the hair is breaking. A protein treatment should be given first by the operator, or a permanent wave made especially for bleached hair may be used. Salons should use the large hair rods where there is bleached or damaged hair, and check the wave pattern every minute.

Question: Can the natural salon products help repair damaged hair, or is their function one of prevention rather than cure?

Answer: Yes, the organic products certainly do repair damaged hair. This is one of the reasons we are so pleased with them and why we suggest a special clinic for damaged hair and the application of both hair and skin preparations for people who are allergic to chemicals.

Perhaps a recent experience of mine will more graphically show the astounding results of these natural beauty aids. One day while making a business contact at a certain beauty salon, I noticed a young patron receiving a hair-bleaching process. The peroxide bleach on her sensitive head had caused blisters to form, some of which were broken and bleeding. Tears of pain were flowing down the customer's cheeks. The color was still not lifting out and was at the "orange stage."

The operator was frantic. The girl had to be back to work in two hours. The operator permitted me to assist her. We thoroughly rinsed off the bleach and applied immediately the new, all-organic bleach I had with me. Made from nature's pure edible foods, this bleach finished the job in fifteen minutes without further pain, actually cutting the remaining bleach time by at least one hour.

Needless to say, that salon owner is now gratefully using this same natural process.

Natural beauty preparations *do* repair as well as prevent damage. With the use of all-organic materials, and the wonderful use of biochemistry, damaged hair can regain glowing healthy beauty.

(Incidentally, according to Jheri Redding, peroxide causes hair color to fade because it leaves a residue. Mr. Redding claims this can be removed by dissolving a little brewers yeast in the rinse water.)

SAFE HAIR RECOLORING

Because many dyes are potentially poisonous and can enter the body via the hair shaft, they may play havoc with health and appearance. One physician eliminates any known source of poisons entering the body. For this reason he absolutely forbids the use of hair dyes.

I have seen women and men with puffy eyes, dark circles, and other unattractive appearance flaws. In nearly every case they had been long-time users of hair dyes.

After noting many cases of damage from certain commercial hair colors, not only to hair, but to health, I asked Mr. Francis for his opinion about hair coloring.

Question: What is tint poisoning?

Answer: It is a term used to designate aniline-derivative poisoning. Aniline, a coal-tar product, is a colorless, poisonous, oily liquid. Its formula is $C_6H_5NH_2$, and it is used in making dyes. The first signs of tint poisoning are the appearance of large, flat bumps, slightly painful; rash around hairline, and swollen ear lobes or eyes. Where there are no external signs, extreme itchiness is felt.

A skin-patch test is required of all persons by federal law. The law states a preliminary test must be given 24 hours before hair is tinted. Many people are allergic to aniline, which tends to be cumulative. Most hair colors contain aniline except "metallic-salts" colors, henna, and of course the pure vegetable hair colors that contain no harmful ingredients at all.

Prolonged use of aniline derivative dyes can cause baldness in some people.

Katherine Pugh, in her book *Baldness: Is It Necessary?* quotes the book *Poisons, Potions, and Profits* by Peter Morell, which states, "Hair dyes probably lead the list as the most dangerous of all the widely used cosmetics. Aniline dyes can be very injurious to those who are sensitive to such chemicals and the damage may be of such varied nature that it would be difficult to trace the dye that caused it."

Medical literature is full of cases of poisoning from hair dyes. Some of the symptoms caused by aniline poisoning include gastro-intestinal problems, severe headaches, nervous disorders, vertigo, and leg weaknesses. Those who value their hair and their health use only the harmless natural products.

In his book *Liver and Cancer*,* Kasper Blond, M.D., reports numerous cases of bladder cancer among aniline dye-workers in Germany, Austria, Great Britain, and the United States.

Some commercial products promise to darken your hair "gradually." They are available in pomade or liquid form, even at stores specializing in health products. Although it may not be true of all of them, the coloring ingredient in the "gradual" colors which I have investigated is lead. Lead can be poisonous, particularly as it slowly accumulates in the body. I have seen people swell around the eye area after one application of hair coloring. Others may not exhibit side effects until the accumulation in the body has reached a high level following many applications.

---

* Kasper Blond, M.D., *Liver and Cancer* (Bristol, England: John Wright and Sons, 1960).

HERBAL HAIR COLORINGS FOR DARK HAIR

Here are some herbal hair colorings which you may wish to try. I cannot state whether they "work" because I do not know anyone who has used them. Since they are made from natural substances, they are presumably safe. As for successful hair recoloring, you will have to experiment for yourself.

Mary Thorne Quelch, in her book of herbal remedies, gives a do-it-yourself formula for darkening hair.

Save left-over tea leaves and tea. In a saucepan, place 1 tablespoon of dried sage leaves and 4 tablespoons of tea leaves. Add water to make 1 pint and simmer for half an hour. Strain and throw away the leaves.

She says, "A little of the infusion to be massaged into the scalp and used to damp the gray hair, four or five times a week. Very gradually the grayness will disappear. After that the use of the infusion once or twice a week will be sufficient. This will do more than darken the hair, it will improve the growth in every way."

Another version of the herbal hair darkener is:

1 ounce sage
1 ounce rosemary
1 pint water

Simmer for 30 minutes and strain. Massage into scalp and gray hair. This is a safe way to darken hair gradually. It is also said to promote growth.

HERBAL COLORINGS FOR BLONDE HAIR

A rinse said to bring out the highlights of blonde hair is made by using 3 or 4 tablespoons of dried camomile flowers to 1 pint of water. Boil from 20 to 30 minutes and strain when cool. Before using, shampoo, since hair must be free from oil. Use the rinse by pouring over the hair while the head is held over the basin. To use the rinse which has dropped into the basin, dip a brush into it and work it into the hair by parting it. Repeat several times.

To prevent a mousy blonde shade, and to keep the hair shiny and keep the scalp free from dandruff, make a shampoo as follows: Boil together ¼ ounce of camomile flowers and ¼ ounce of quassia chips 10 to 15 minutes in enough water to make a reasonable amount of rinse. Use once or twice a week.

For hair which was once blonde, a woman gave me a folk remedy which had come down through three generations in her family: ten grams each of licorice root and oat straw. Add a pinch of saffron. Cover with water and boil to make an infusion. Strain and use as a rinse which is allowed to soak into the hair, but not washed off until the next shampoo.

There are further herbal colorings suggested in a free leaflet which is available from Indiana Botanic Gardens, Hammond, Indiana 46325. They also supply the necessary herbs.

Although the formulas in this leaflet are far safer than the dangerous aniline commercial dyes, still, they require a great deal of experimentation to produce the correct shade. Henna, used for red hair and in some herbal colorings, is extremely tricky. It can, in inexpert hands, produce bizarre colors. For example, plain henna used on white hair can turn it flaming orange or pink. If hair has been previously dyed with chemicals; if your scalp is irritated; or if you are suffering from a skin disturbance, do not use it at all. In my opinion, it is better to use the "Living Colors" which have been safely and successfully used in thousands of cases. Mr. Francis will describe them below.

Ask your salon to order these colors. You can also order them from health stores, for coloring your own hair at home.

Dyed hair often gives away its secret because it is *all one color*. Naturally colored hair is never a single color. Look at a child's hair under the revealing light of sunshine. No matter what the color, it is made up of hundreds of different shades. This produces highlights, and, in turn, beauty. Strive for this effect when you are coloring your own hair.

To return to Mr. Francis, I asked his opinion on hair colorings.

Question: Is a safe hair coloring available?

Answer: There is recent extraordinary achievement in hair coloring. It is unlike any previous commercial product. There are 12 basic chromatic shades which can be expanded to 48 or more shades by means of a dilution of a specially blended oil. It brings out the highlights of the hair without producing a rough, porous, or tinted feel. If one prefers to tone down reddish highlights, a "drabber" is added. This will leave the hair strong and healthy. Any beauty operator can quickly learn to use it. It can even be a do-it-yourself project.

Because some people are allergic even to some foods, a patch test, and other rules for handling these colors (they are listed in the directions) are sensible precautions. However, these nonallergic hair colors may be safely used.

Out of the thousands of satisfied users we have had only two that had slight reactions and this was only for the first time. Both women, who were previously allergic to all other brands of tints, had the required 24-hour patch test behind the ear which showed negative. Yet when the tint was applied they showed some reaction.

Since the natural tints, including the developer, are created from oranges, tomatoes, cucumbers, and other vegetable substances instead of dangerous chemicals like aniline derivatives or metallic salts, we do not have to be concerned about synthetic chemical reactions, but because some people are allergic to certain fruits or vegetables, a patch test is required for the first time.

In the case of these two ladies, a little sleuthing indicated that their systems were not compatible to one or two things: (1) A possible reaction to henna, which is a hair coloring used during Cleopatra's day and is from a shrub cultivated since ancient times in Egypt. It is used in the red and brown shades of the natural tints; (2) An incompatibility of the particles of the previous chemical color remaining in the skin to the natural tint. It has been found that even women who have stopped tinting their hair with aniline dyes still have an accumulation of aniline in their systems and several years may go by before these particles are eliminated. At any time their presence could trigger a reaction.

Why doesn't this happen all the time to others switching from the synthetic to the natural products? Simply this: A third chemical factor enters the picture—the highly sensitized chemical combination in the individual who couldn't handle the aniline dyes in the first place, let alone the turmoil between the two. Once a previous tint was cleared off the hair and scalp, both women have had no problems whatsoever with subsequent tintings which left the hair soft and natural and the scalp free of the "weeping" eczema they had suffered with for years when using aniline dyes.

One customer wrote me, "The natural hair coloring is particularly kind to soft, fine hair and to permanents. My hair was restored after being severely damaged by one of the best-known hair tints, advertised nationally."

Question: Is this coloring process only for women, or can men use it, too?

Answer: Hair color, or any "aid" that wisely and health-fully improves one's appearance and sense of well-being should never be limited to a certain sex or age group. Men certainly have every right to take personal pride in how they look and to take advantage of advances made available for this purpose. To be well-groomed enhances masculinity.

There is no reason why the men cannot color their own hair if they desire.

To do so, the hair should be thoroughly washed. The best shampoos are of organic material found at most health-food stores. No regular bar soap, please. It ruins the hair, destroying the natural and necessary protective acid mantle on the scalp. If shampoos other than the organic are used, get nondetergent ones, but be sure to use a vinegar or lemon-and-water rinse afterward.

After lathering, scrub scalp gently with scalp brush to cleanse properly. If hair dressing has not been used, hair may be colored without washing. To color, simply mix 1 part color and 1 part developer in an applicator bottle, shake, and apply a few drops at a time and comb through until the entire hair is moist (not drippy). Let set the length of time required. Next clean skin and ears with wash cloth, using straight shampoo. Then wash hair, and comb.

If one prefers the color change to be gradual, so it isn't obvious, color should be left on for only 10 minutes the first time, about 15 minutes the second time, and for the full 25 minutes the third time.

Question: Incidentally, do you recommend hair sprays?

Answer: There are many hair sprays on the market, but what appears to be a bargain may not be. Everyone should realize that most of the so-called bargains contain varnish, shellac, or lacquer emulsified in water with a little perfume added, perhaps along with a little lanolin. The knowledge-able individual knows this type of product is dangerous, but unfortunately the general public does not.

The lacquer-based sprays immediately seal the skin pores, sealing in the sebaceous and waste materials, causing both the pores and the hair roots to become impacted. This interferes with the normal skin functions and can stunt hair growth. It also causes itching, scaling, and cysts.

It is true that hair sprays are convenient, but one should

not compromise the health of hair and scalp for the sake of convenience—nor is it necessary. Those who feel the need of hair sprays can obtain them from most health stores and from beauty salons which carry natural beauty products.

We know of an excellent hair spray, and advise its use in salons along with the natural permanents and tints. It is an all-natural, organic spray made from the orange-peel oil of organically grown oranges, mixed with soybean oil for the protein element. Bottled in a nontoxic container, it does an excellent job of holding the hair in place. Its delightful, light fragrance resembles that of orange blossoms. On the scalp it leaves breathing spots for the skin. We think you will agree with us that it is a wonderful product.

Question: Why don't more beauty salons use the type of natural and healthful beauty products you have described?

Answer: Remember, your beauty operator wants the best for you and does not manufacture the chemical solutions he must use in his business. He merely uses what is available. Let's all pass the word around so that everyone will have the opportunity for healthful, safe beauty. Every salon could use natural sprays, shampoos, permanents, and hair colorings. They may not know about them. Call your local beauty operator and inquire about them. Let your operator know that you want the very best. You can be instrumental in encouraging your local salons to carry these safe products.

NUTRITIONAL HAIR RECOLORING

Is it possible to return graying hair to its natural color through nutrition alone? We have been considering some safe hair dyes, but is it really possible to get rid of your gray hair permanently so that you don't have to dye, rinse, or touch up at all? Some people have done it, and are doing it. I do want to make it clear, however, that the cause of gray hair is not always the same for everyone, hence the treatment may be different. Also, most people who have had hair color return to its normal shade report that it takes time. Usually they get so excited, though, that the very fact that they see progress brings its own reward. One caution: a slap-dash method, or a now-and-then, hit-or-miss approach will not work. You must be *thorough* and *consistent!* And it is only fair to tell you that, though some have changed their hair color back to normal, there are others who did not. Perhaps it was due to heredity, perhaps to the wrong combination of nutrients. Yet the very fact that some people are having success means that it is worth trying, don't you think?

Adelle Davis says, "Probably every nutrient influences the health of the hair.

"Adequate amounts of iron, copper, iodine, and the following B vitamins are essential in maintaining the natural color of the hair: pantothenic acid (calcium pantothenate), PABA, folic acid, and inositol. Gray hair at any age, particularly prematurely gray hair, probably indicates a deficiency of one or more of these nutrients.

"The natural color of gray hair has sometimes been restored by an adequate intake of all the anti-gray-hair vitamins. The most marked results in restoration of color of gray hair have come from a liberal use of natural foods supplying B vitamins: brewers yeast, blackstrap molasses, wheat germ, rice polishings, liver, and yogurt.

"When liberal amounts of yogurt are taken daily, the yogurt bacteria growing in the intestinal tract apparently synthesize or produce the B vitamin inositol, and other anti-gray-hair vitamins. The richest sources of inositol are whole wheat breads, brewers yeast, blackstrap molasses, and wheat germ."

WHAT CAUSES GRAY HAIR?

Some causes of gray hair may not yet be known; others are established: stress, poor circulation to the scalp, anemia, lack of iodine or copper in the diet; lack of certain B vitamins; a lack of unsaturated fatty acids, malnourished glands which need certain raw materials to produce color and, lastly, heredity.

Dr. Agnes Fay Morgan, dean of nutrition researchers at the University of California at Berkeley, found that with animals a deficient diet produced malfunctioning glands, followed by loss of hair color. Upon supplying the missing nutrients to the animals, the glands were repaired for the most part, and the hair turned back to its normal color. All of this was established by autopsies on the animals. The major vitamin Dr. Morgan used was pantothenic acid, a B vitamin. An M.D. in Boston, Dr. Benjamin Sieve, gave another B vitamin, PABA, to 300 of his patients with graying hair. The patients were of both sexes and ranged in age from sixteen to seventy-four. They had been gray from two years to twenty-four years. Changes in their hair was usually noted within the first five weeks. Hair lustre and health improved, too.

When pantothenic acid (a B vitamin), used by Dr. Morgan, is absent from an otherwise adequate diet for animals (which is one of the ways we learn what humans also need) the animals' hair turns gray, anemia and eczema appear, the animals appear old before their time, even when they are young. They also develop stomach and duodenal ulcers, and damage to heart muscles, liver, kidney, thyroid and sex glands. In two groups of cocker spaniels, those which were not fed pantothenic acid appeared old, droopy, and without energy. The hair became gray. When pantothenic acid was restored to their diet it restored, somewhat, their youthful appearance. The animals which had never been deprived of this vitamin had sleek fur of beautiful color, were full of pep, youth, and vitality. Although pantothenic acid may not be the example, there are instances in which taking high amounts of a single B vitamin alone has caused disturbances because, strangely, giving too much of one has been known to create a deficiency of another. However, pantothenic acid can be taken with the full vitamin-B complex—just to be on the safe side. Foods rich in pantothenic acid are: liver, brewers yeast, rice polishings, wheat germ, soybeans, peanuts, egg yolk and, to some extent, whole grains. When you eat white bread, you are getting no pantothenic acid at all because refining of flour removes it.

I have before-and-after pictures of a handsome world-champion wrestler who has nutritionally recolored his hair. He added to a diet which included *everything* needed nutritionally, a combination of blackstrap molasses, natural honey, and apple cider vinegar, which he uses as a beverage daily. Every morning he combines two tablespoons each of this mixture to his drinking water. He says that it took about a year for complete recoloring of his hair. I can vouch for this story, since I met him personally several years ago.

I recently saw this man again and his hair still remains beautiful, dark, and without a single strand of gray. I asked him if he had ever retested his beverage formula to be *sure* it was responsible for recoloring his hair. He answered, "Yes. I gave it up for two months. My hair started graying and then falling. When I resumed taking the mixture, the dark color returned and the falling stopped. I also learned that, for some reason, honey was necessary, too."

The ingredients in this mixture contain vitamins and minerals, already mentioned in connection with hair-coloring experiments. Blackstrap is especially high in copper and iron. In fact, several nutrition researchers believe that copper is the most effective element of all for reversing gray hair in humans. Vinegar provides acid (as well as potassium) to help the assimilation of minerals. But let me repeat: the concoction which this man drinks is not the *only* nutritional addition to his diet. He eats only highly nutritious food and takes every vitamin, mineral, and other nutritional substance known, as well. This program returned him to perfect health after doctors had given him up to die. The addition of the blackstrap-honey-vinegar mixture was only one part of the complete nutritional program responsible for his rehabilitation. When I use this formula, as I do from time to time to help correct two or three gray spots which appeared in my hair in my early thirties, I always notice the same results. First the color begins to reappear in the hairs on my arms; next a deepening of color is noticeable in my eyebrows. Finally, it shows up on my scalp. If I give it up for long, as I must when I travel, the color gradually recedes in all areas.

One woman has recolored her hair through a certain breakfast food. She developed this breakfast food herself after she had a child twenty years after marriage. Her hair was beginning to gray and she decided she didn't want to look like her daughter's grandmother. So she snipped off a lock of her hair, took it to her doctor to keep as a record, then began to experiment. The experiment worked and the doctor's periodic collection of locks of hair, which showed changed color along the way, is proof that it worked.

In order to develop the breakfast food, after reading everything she could find on the recoloring attributes of various foods, she came up with a formula which she will not divulge. In general, it includes such things as organically grown nuts, figs, dates, herbs, alfalfa, kelp, powdered bone meal, mung bean sprouts and many other things. All of the ingredients are used raw to preserve the precious enzymes. The inventor of this breakfast food has been eating it for several years now and her hair has returned to its original color. I have before-and-after samples as proof. The exact formula for this breakfast food is not available.

Certainly nutritional hair coloring is worth a try. I hope it works for you, too.

19 Stay Slim Comfortably

Nearly everybody is overweight. Before I tell you how to overcome it, let's find out what causes it. There are probably two basic causes: physical hunger and emotional hunger.

Because so many people have nutritional "hidden hunger" or are deficient in nutrients necessary to keep their bodies in repair, the wisdom of their bodies probably keeps gnawing at their appetites, seeking a sufficient supply of necessary nutrients. Because so much food, through refining and processing, now contains so little nutrients, one has to eat more in order to make up for these "empty calories." This is why vitamins and minerals, added to a good diet, are so helpful; they prevent eating so much bulk in order to obtain the correct amount of nutrition.

Emotional stress complicates the problem. As tensions accumulate, some people turn to food as a prop. Others use drugs, alcohol, and tobacco.

Whether the cause is nutritional or emotional, it is clear that overweights are seeking some deeper form of satisfaction.

EMOTIONAL HELPS

People eat from loneliness, depression, hurt feelings, resentment, or from feeling unloved, unwanted. They eat to pamper or console themselves. Boredom is another cause of overweight. I know one woman who has absolutely no interest in life except food. The minute she wakens in the morning, she begins to plan what she is going to eat. She is one of those people who truly live to eat because she has not found anything else to live for. Taking a course, learning a craft, acting as a hospital volunteer, reading to shut-ins or merely talking with them to cheer them up—any one of a dozen good work projects would take this woman's mind off food and help her to a much-needed loss of 40 pounds.

The first step a compulsive eater should take is to face himself honestly and figure out why he overeats. This is half the battle. Then by substituting constructive other things for food, he finds eating nonstop is no longer necessary. If you do overeat because you are lonely, remember you can dine with the most famous people in the world, either by radio, television or books. Listening to, watching, or reading about someone else at mealtime will help you feel less alone and less in need of a second helping of food to console you.

Sometimes one small glass of wine sipped with an evening meal gives comfort and something pleasurable to look forward to during the day. It provides both nutritional and psychological value.

Dr. Salvatore P. Lucia, a university professor of preventive medicine, believes the ancient physicians, Hippocrates, Galen and others, were right in using wine as medicine. He says, "Wine has nutritional value due to its content of B vitamins and minerals: potassium, magnesium, sodium, calcium, iron, and phosphorus." Dr. Lucia feels wine stimulates better digestion. Aside from the nutritional content, dry wine has provided much-needed acid for many people. Dr. Lucia feels that wine as a medicine, as well as a psychological lift before or with the evening meal, is good for the aging. He says, "The gentle sedation produced by wine can often dispel the fears and anxieties of old age and at the same time ensure restful sleep."

A 3-ounce glass of dry wine taken *before* a meal stimulates appetite. Medical studies have found that a 3-ounce glass of dry wine taken *with* a meal helps food to be better assimilated and is also an aid in reducing. In either case, however, the rules must be followed: only 3 ounces of *dry* wine is allowed. Sweet wine adds calories.

Even the Bible recommends wine in moderation: First Timothy 5:23 states, "Drink no longer water, but use a little wine for thy stomach's sake and thine often infirmities."

But Ephesians 5:18 cautions: "And be not drunk with wine; but be filled with the Spirit."

So the secret is to drink a very little wine. Carried to excess it has caused worse cases of drunkenness than hard liquor. You have to know when to stop. Don't overdo it and take "just one more!" Limit yourself to slowly sipping a 3-ounce glass of dry wine on the rocks, which dilutes it.

During a reducing program, the cocktail hour is the cause of most backsliding. A person sips a cocktail and one of two things happens: either he keeps on drinking or he becomes ravenously hungry and stows away hors d'oeuvres by the plateful. Often these are more fattening than the alcohol.

One woman said that she and her husband looked forward to the cocktail hour with enthusiasm, but she discovered it was conviviality and the glass, not the content, which created the pleasure of the "happy hour." She found that tomato juice or plain soda water was just as relaxing, and that raw vegetables served as hors d'oeuvres are practically zero in calories.

Cary Grant has noted that a woman who neither smokes nor drinks seems to have a better complexion than those who do. Arlene Dahl, model, movie star, and beauty columnist, adds, "Most dermatologists agree with him. They consider alcoholic beverages skin-poison. Alcohol is as harmful for the figure as it is for the face."

Some experts believe that alcohol causes water storage, thus adds weight.

BE CAREFUL OF SWEETS

Children have long been rewarded with "sweets" for some type of suffering. Doctors, unfortunately, may give a child a lollipop after an inoculation; even some dentists offer sweets (which cause more cavities) after a painful siege in the dentist's chair. As a carry-over from childhood, overweights follow the same principle: They "reward" themselves with sweets to compensate for an unhappy experience or state of mind.

Sweets cause overweight.

Dee Wells, writing about Queen Elizabeth II, says, "Queen Elizabeth has shed about 25 pounds. The royal women have always had a strong liking for candy, thickly iced cakes, and cream-laden puddings. But because she must appear at her best as well as feel her best, the royal diet includes a total ban on alcohol, candy, pastry, dessert, nuts, and even jam and marmalade. The Queen is allowed only four teacups of liquid a day, no fried food."

WHEN TO GO ON A DIET

Reducing should not be undertaken during times of stress. Your body needs all the help it can get. Worry over money, domestic affairs, or a lost job is strain enough. One writer tells of another writer who went on a diet while he was trying to finish a book by deadline time. He reached the point where his mind became stuck on baked potatoes and apple pie instead of his book, and he had to postpone the diet until the book was finished.

Incidentally, sometimes during dieting, you become obsessed with a longing for a fattening dish. You can't seem to think about anything less caloric. If this hits you, try the dish, or that gooey dessert—whatever it is. But if the first bite doesn't taste as good as you expected, don't take any more. As you wean yourself from sweet foods, you will reach the point where they may *look* good but they no longer *taste* good.

There are days when you should be eating, psychologically. It would cause depression if you didn't. On the other hand, there are days when you wake up rarin' to go and you are willing to do *anything* to get rid of those unwanted pounds. Move with the tide.

And by all means, diet in secret. There is something perverse about anyone who watches another one diet. The nondieter will try to bully you into eating this "just once" (which may be your undoing) or will tell you confidentially that you would look better if you didn't diet. Perhaps it's jealousy on the part of the nondieter, but for your own protection, just keep the whole thing to yourself.

WHY YOU MAY NOT LOSE WEIGHT ON A REDUCING DIET

Much overweight is caused by water retention. This is one reason why you often reach a plateau in weight loss. It is probably nature's protective system to give your body a chance to catch its breath before more weight disappears. One physician says, "Water is produced as fat is burned.

For every pound of fat burned, in addition to what you drink, 1¼ pounds of water are produced in your body. This is nature's compensation to the body, but it can be mighty discouraging to the dieter."

Some doctors prescribe a diuretic to get rid of the water, but it is risky business, since the diuretic could act quickly, eliminating many pounds (of water) within days, even hours, washing away water-soluble vitamins and other body-protecting nutrients. Dr. Harry C. Shirkey, of Samford University, Birmingham, Alabama, points out that in using diuretic drugs, vitamins and essential body chemicals are lost as well as weight. The result: a thinner person with metabolic disturbances.

Taking vitamin B-6 is a much safer way to regulate abnormal water storage.

Some people complain that when they start on a reducing diet they actually gain instead of lose. Joseph Lederman, M.D., in his book* explains why.

He says, "On a low calorie diet the loss of weight occurs in a staircase pattern. First, excess body fat is burned. About four and a half ounces of water are formed and stored within the tissues for every ounce of this burned fat. Thus the dieter may not lose weight immediately; in fact he may gain several pounds for a brief period. But soon there is a change in the water tissue balance, the excess of fluid eliminated, and the scale shows a weight loss."

THE EDIBLE-FAT CONTROVERSY

So many misstatements or premature warnings have been issued against eating fat that people have become panicky about it. Many won't buy anything but skim milk. Others are afraid to eat an egg. Even doctors are misinformed on this subject. Because dairy foods contain cholesterol, many people (including many doctors who have not had time to read the latest findings) are unaware that the body manufactures cholesterol whether you eat it or not. Cholesterol is needed to help your glands. (Lecithin can be used to dissolve cholesterol in the body.)

A fat-free diet is not only out of date, it is actually dangerous. A Bucknell University study showed that a fat-

* Be Fit, Not Fat (St. Louis: Education Publishers, Inc., 1962).

free diet can cause gallstones in experimental animals. A gall bladder needs fat to work properly. Without it, it becomes sluggish.

Adelle Davis reported that people on fat-free diets became overweight with swollen legs, ankles, and thighs. When they added two tablespoons of salad oil daily, they lost *pounds*. One Powers model was unable to reduce *until she added fat*, in the form of oils, to her diet.

Calories from fat and protein are burned up by the body to provide energy and are not stored as fat.

One friend of mine who was both overweight and addicted to sweets began to substitute fats for sweets. She took a tablespoon of oil in juice, or a tablespoonful of natural peanut butter whenever she had "that empty feeling." She told me facetiously, "I haven't been hungry since!"

There has been a lot of fuss about the "Calories Don't Count" diet. This is merely a high-protein, high-fat, low-carbohydrate diet discovered by Stefansson, the anthropologist. It has been slightly varied and called a lot of other names such as "The Drinking Man's Diet" (plus alcohol), the "Martinis and Whipped Cream Diet," the "Air Force Diet," the "Eat Fat and Stay Slim Diet," the "Du Pont Diet" (because it was tested on workers in the Du Pont plant) and later called "The Holiday Diet" because it appeared in *Holiday* magazine.

The reason that the book about the calories-don't-count diet was challenged is that only a few safflower oil *capsules* were recommended. Any type of unsaturated oils, in order to be effective, should be used in larger amounts than are found in a few capsules.

Frankly, I am getting weary about all the fuss against this type of diet. Stefansson, before he died in his late eighties, was one of my dear friends, and I believe that I discussed this diet with him as throroughly as any nutrition reporter did. Here is the story he told me which led to the "Stefansson Diet," bandied about under so many names:

He and a companion were traveling on foot in the Arctic carrying rations of caribou meat (lean) and seal oil (fat). The supply of seal oil was eventually exhausted, leaving them with only lean meat. Immediately the two men became headachy and suffered from diarrhea to such a degree that they were afraid they were going to die. Luckily an Eskimo passed them and shared his supply of seal oil with the two white men. Within a few hours after taking the oil, the headaches stopped and the diarrhea disappeared.

Stefansson told me, "That taught me a lesson. I never was on a fat-free diet the rest of my life." When writers stated that he was living on a high-protein diet, as he had in the Arctic, he said, indignantly, "I am *not* living on a high-protein diet. I am eating a *high-fat* diet."

Though the Eskimos were high-protein eaters, they were essentially high-fat eaters. Eighty per cent of their calories came from fat. Both Stefansson and the Eskimos felt wonderful on this high-fat diet and were never overweight.

In fact, W. A. Pennington, M.D., found that of the twenty men and women tested in the Du Pont Corporation, all lost weight on this same general diet even though the total calorie intake was unrestricted. (This explains the name "calories-don't count.") The dieters ate about 3,000 calories a day, but extra meat and fat were allowed those who wanted more. No one was hungry; all reported a great sense of well-being.

The reason why Dr. Herman Taller wrote *Calories Don't Count* is because he himself had been overweight for many years and had tried every known reducing diet without success. After learning about the Stefansson Diet, he added 3 ounces of liquid vegetable oil (it happened to be safflower-oil) to his daily diet and for the first time in his life his weight became normal. Then he tried it on his patients. They, too, succeeded in losing weight.

About ten different investigators have tested the diet and each has christened it with a new name. McGill University in Canada tried it on volunteers who had had no success with all previous methods of reducing. It worked; the volunteers were never hungry; and after losing from 10 to 40 pounds, those who were still living on the diet two years later had not gained back their weight.

George Watson, a researcher from the University of California, believes that a *little* carbohydrate is necessary in this type of diet to help burn fat and produce a greater feeling of well-being. According to one nutritional physician, it should be a *natural* carbohydrate, however: a baked potato, whole brown rice, whole grain bread or cereal, fruit, vegetables, or a salad. He believes it should not be white sugar, white flour or other processed foods, or rich desserts.

WHAT ABOUT "LOW-CALORIE" FOODS?

Another misconception about dieting is artificial sweeteners, especially calcium cyclamate and sodium cyclamate. Franklin Bicknell, M.D., a consulting physician in London, warns: "All artificial sweeteners cause general toxicity in animals. One variety causes liver tumors, another kidney damage, and still another, diarrhea."

Still more serious, a Japanese physician, Dr. Ryozo Tanaka of the Iwate Medical College, has conducted a study with mice, with the shocking results that the sodium and calcium cyclamates either killed the unborn or, in many cases, caused birth defects similar to those produced by thalidomide.

Many doctors in America are becoming concerned about the effects of these artificial sweeteners on health as they learn of their hazards. Consumption of the sweeteners has nearly tripled since 1960 and they are appearing in canned and processed foods as well as soft drinks, fruit juice, fruits, syrups, toppings, desserts, cookies, cakes and mixes; even canned Chinese dinners are riddled with them. Why? Artificial sweeteners are big business. Every manufacturer wants to get on the money bandwagon, as every consumer seems to think the artificial sweeteners are the "open sesame" to reducing. Far from it! Doctors solemnly warn that only the *right diet* can reduce weight. The few calories missing in a low-calorie food or beverage is not enough to cause weight loss and prevent overweight. The sweeteners, particularly the cyclamates, are considered potentially dangerous by those who have tested them thoroughly and reported the results honestly. Both the public and the manufacturers would rather not listen.

To avoid them, read your labels before buying. For safety, use natural sweetening such as honey, instead. A small amount will not be a threat to your weight.

ARE REDUCING DRUGS SAFE?

Richard Carter, in his book,* writes that if eating is a compulsion, appetite depressants are of little use. Mr. Carter warns that the drugs increase the pulse rate, make

* Richard Carter, *Your Food and Your Health* (New York: Harper & Row, 1964).

some patients shaky, and act only as a chemical crutch. When reducers give them up, they usually gain back the lost pounds. The AMA has issued even more serious warnings against reducing drugs.

Henry Brill, M.D., a psychiatrist, says, "Overuse can result in excessive beating of the heart, hypertension (high blood pressure), nervousness, emotional tension, and hallucinations."

James B. Landis, of Smith, Kline and French Laboratories, warns that even pep pills can affect the appetite center of the brain and become a dangerous crutch. He says, "A psychosis resembling schizophrenia can develop on large, excessive, daily doses."

The American Medical Association believes that diet pills, including thyroid, hormones, digitalis, and diuretics, not only won't work, but may be extremely dangerous. At least sixty deaths have been attributable to diet pills.

DOES EXERCISE HELP REDUCERS?

Dr. Jean Mayer, professor of nutrition at Harvard University, believes that exercise is a *must* for reducers. He says that in many cases it is not the food alone that makes people overweight. Fatties eat more than they burn off. An extra Martini per day means 10 pounds of fat per year. An extra half-sandwich could be burned off with a 20-minute walk each day. Dr. Mayer adds, "The fat man's biggest single villain is lack of exercise. Nor does the American woman walk 10 miles a day in her home; it is usually more like 250 yards."

Dr. Mayer believes exercise in spurts is not enough; his regimen for fat people is regular exercise, good nutrition, and persistence.

Richard Carter agrees. He says that young people usually don't need to lose weight; they are active. However, active people who become less active in middle years usually do not automatically reduce their food intake to match. This is why they gain weight.

BEWARE OF FASTING TO LOSE WEIGHT

One nutritional M.D. told me, "I wish you could see the delayed results of fad diets in the tissues of my patients. Fad diets include only a few nutrients daily (i.e., a banana diet, a cottage cheese diet). During a fad or partial diet, the body is not receiving all the repair material it needs; it feeds on itself, and tissues, organs, and glands pay the price later. The body. needs *every* nutrient *every* day."

Fasting without the inclusion of the missing nutrients can play havoc with health. *The American Journal of Clinical Nutrition* (July, 1967), reporting the work of five researchers, stated, "During complete fasting, significant metabolic stresses will develop and may eventually result in serious abnormalities. Under fasting conditions both fat and protein body stores are being utilized as sources of energy. . . . Complete fasting without mineral and vitamin supplements should not be recommended. . . . Otherwise a severe stress could eventually lead to greatly impaired mental [ability] and physical inefficiency."

Needless to say, fasting should be done only under the supervision of a qualified physician.

There is much agreement from other specialists on the danger of total and prolonged fasting. The National Arthritis Institute, Bethesda, Maryland, found that fasting created a deficiency of riboflavin—a B vitamin necessary for good vision and skin. The Department of Medicine at the University of Virginia Medical School found that prolonged fasting produced blood sugar tolerance curves typical of "starvation diabetes." A Danish study of people who were reducing by total fasting plus vitamins stated, "Total fasting is considered unsuitable for patients with arthritis, gout or heart disease."

Lothar Gottlieb Tirala, M.D., Ph.D., of Wiesbaden, Germany, writing in *Let's Live* (November, 1966), says, "It is a delusion to believe that through prolonged fasting-cures, lasting for weeks, diseases can be cured. Those who attempt a cure by drastic fasting may cause great harm.

"Persons undergoing such starvation cures in health resorts, receiving only water for two to four weeks, are damaging their health considerably. . . . The muscles waste away, and a great number of toxic substances appear in the urine and blood. The fasting person consumes his own muscles, which means he virtually eats himself. When a man of normal weight is on drastic fasting, receiving only water or fruit juices, he will, after a few days, use up 150 grams of his muscle flesh daily.

"The lay practitioners believe wrongly that through enforced fasting latent toxic substances are removed from the body, because toxins appear in the patient's urine. This is a grave error; *the toxic substances are produced* by the fasting. The serum proteins which accomplish water transportation in the body disappear rapidly. The water remains in the connective tissues of the underskin and edema sets in on the legs and face."

Dr. Tirala lists other deterioration resulting from such fasting: intestines cease to function; edema of the stomach and intestines occurs, producing gastro-intestinal disorders; gamma globulins and essential hormones disappear from the blood; the ovaries and testes stop functioning; and mental capacity and judgment deteriorate as a result of low blood sugar. Even in the first week, he says, depression, apathy, psychosis, even hallucinations are noticeable. He warns, *"There is no chronic disease which can be cured by fasting.* A mild fasting for two to three weeks is indicated only in cases of acute inflammation of kidneys and acute pancreatitis. . . . With the slight shock to the vegetative system from a three-day-long raw food diet, the edema of a patient suffering from heart disease can be drained away quickly and easily, but woe betide him if one dare to treat such a person by fasting."

HOW TO LOSE WEIGHT SAFELY

Dr. Brady, in his syndicated newspaper column, writes: "Many a woman has learned the hard way how wrinkles come from irrational, unphysiological reduction dieting or rapid reduction by the use of drugs, salts, or other physic, which impairs nutrition. And many a girl acquires wrinkles prematurely by restricting her diet unwisely in the effort to keep underweight."

How you eat is as important as what you eat. The nibble diet is one of the safe keys to weight reduction. Your stomach is elastic, like a balloon. At Thanksgiving and Christmas, for example, you groan, "I feel stuffed, but after all Thanksgiving (or Christmas) comes only once a year."

True, but here is what happens to your stomach. Having been stretched with all the unaccustomed food, it remains *stretched*. So the next day your stomach demands the same amount of food to satisfy its new dimensions.

Conversely, this is why the first three days of a diet are so uncomfortable. Your stomach is demanding more food, while you are trying to cut down and ignore its demand. Everyone who has ever stuck out the first three days of dieting admits they are the hardest. After that it is a cinch. Your stomach has shrunk and no longer demands so much food.

On-again, off-again dieting upsets the body balance, too. Body controls get out of kilter and can eventually cause real trouble. One answer is the nibble diet. Eating in small amounts many times a day controls hunger, stores up your energy, and keeps your stomach capacity small. Though you may nibble all day, this does not mean you can eat *more;* it merely means that you divide the same amount of food found in "three squares" into smaller portions. By eating oftener, you put less strain on your digestion as well as on your disposition.

A study conducted by Czech researchers on 450 men found that those who ate two big meals a day gained more weight than those who ate four or five meals a day plus snacks in between. The scientists decided that the reason is that the person who eats frequent small meals can burn up his food as fast as he eats it. In big meals, however, he stores up the excess as fat.

Ben Weider, writing in *Vigor* magazine, tells how the nibble diet helped him. He says, "Try the nibble diet for yourself for one week. See how it works for you. Concentrate on high-protein foods, such as lean meats, fish, poultry, eggs, and skim milk. Then supplement these with low-carbohydrate vegetables such as broccoli, spinach, asparagus, celery, and lettuce. Be sure to eat a little fresh fruit every day and keep your bread down to a minimum, eating, all-in-all, only very small amounts of food several times during the day.

"Eat only until you are no longer hungry and no more! This may take quite a bit of self-training, since you have been eating on the three-day plan for your entire life, and probably more than half the food you consume is eaten not to satisfy hunger, but merely out of habit.

"I have been on this diet myself for the past 10 days and have found everything wonderfully satisfying. I eat raw vegetables much of the time, and cold chicken or turkey every other day. At supper time I eat a hot meal, along with the rest of the family—but I eat *very, very little of everything.*

"Best of all, I have lost 4 pounds in these last 10 days, and I have never once felt the pangs of hunger!"

A University of Chicago study showed that eating

the heavy meal at night causes a weight gain. Harvey D. Smith, M.D., a reducing specialist, believes that the heavier a person gets, the more carbohydrates he craves (which makes him still heavier); and that many people eat at the wrong time. He says:

"I have many patients who eat only 800 or 900 calories, yet who are gaining weight. I can put them on 1,500 calories and have them lose weight with a more balanced diet, taking most of the calories at breakfast and lunch. That's the secret of good dieting: to take in the same amount or more calories, yet lose weight—it depends largely on *when* you eat.

"Breakfast should provide approximately 40 percent of the caloric intake, balanced between carbohydrates and protein; lunch, 40 percent; supper should not exceed 20 percent of the daily intake.

" 'But doctor, I can't eat a thing for breakfast; then I get very hungry later in the day.'

"This is typical of the many excuses I hear from patients explaining why they can't lose weight 'no matter how they try.' Most people eat practically nothing at breakfast—and then burn up the day's energy. At evening meals, they eat many calories, after which they sit around doing nothing. If they would reverse this procedure and eat more calories of the normal breakfast-type food in the morning and less in the evening, 90 percent of overweight people would help themselves."*

A NEW WAY TO DIET EASILY

A unique method of reducing is presented by Elizabeth Keyes, in her little book, *How to Win the Losing Fight*.** I don't want to give away the entire secret, but I will give you the gist of it and you can later read the rest for yourself. Mrs. Keyes had a weight problem from childhood. She tried everything. Nothing worked. Finally she learned about this special method in which you can eat as much as you wish, as often as you wish, and get thin. Her first trial was rewarded by several pounds' loss in the first week.

Elizabeth Keyes is the founder of "Overweight Overcomers International" (OOI). I looked over some Christmas cards written to her by members of one of these

* *Family Weekly*, Feb. 9, 1969.
** Gentle Living Publications, 2168 South Lafayette, Denver, Colorado 80201.

volunteer groups who had read her book. One woman had lost 65 pounds since the first of the year. Others had lost varying amounts according to their needs and wishes. All were ecstatic about the method.

In general, Mrs. Keyes says, the method is based on the fact that all overweight people are gulpers. They swallow their food whole and, not being satisfied, take one helping after another. Here is her method: Take a bite the size of a pea. Put your fork down and relax while you chew it. Savor and enjoy every shred of flavor in that bite. When the bite has literally melted away in your mouth, then, and only then, take another bite and repeat the process. You will be amazed at how soon your appetite will disappear and how little food you will have eaten.

She tells of a woman who tried it. This woman was brought to a demonstration breakfast attended by fifty women, members of OOI. The overweight woman was evidently dragged there by a determined relative who wanted her to reduce. Mrs. Overweight was greeted by Mrs. Keyes and told she could order anything, absolutely anything she wished for her breakfast. Defiantly she ordered hot cakes and syrup, butter, bacon and eggs, coffee with cream and sugar. When it was served to her, she fell to with gusto.

Mrs. Keyes said, "Wait! Cut off only a small bite, like this."

The woman complained, "I can't even taste that. It's so tiny I wouldn't know when I swallowed it."

But she followed directions. She held it in her mouth, tasted it, sucked the flavor between her tongue and palate, closed her eyes, and enjoyed it to the fullest.

Mrs. Keyes then turned her attention to others around the table. She said, "After a while I noticed that my lady was sitting back, staring at her plate with a strange expression. She had eaten less than one-fourth of the cakes, one half-slice of the four slices of bacon, and had not touched the eggs.

" 'Is something wrong?' I asked.

"She shoved the plate back. 'Yes. It doesn't taste like I thought it would. In fact, it tastes awful. I've never been so disappointed in my life.' "

Mrs. Keyes coaxed her to take a little more. The woman said, "I don't want any more of the stuff. It would make me sick if I had to eat it."

Laughter went around the table as the other women cried, "She's converted."

Later that day the woman stopped Mrs. Keyes on the street. She said, "Do you know, I'm not hungry *yet*. Do you suppose something is wrong with me?"

Mrs. Keyes assured her that for the first time in years she was on the right track.

Mrs. Keyes combines good nutrition with "gentle eating," as she calls it. By using proper foods and this method of thoroughly tasting, enjoying, and chewing each bite, you will soon eat only half of your former portions, have better digestion, and lose weight without discomfort.

Frank B. Lachle, a chemist and nutrition adviser, sums up the ideal reducing diet. He says, "If we supply our bodies with the total ingredients required for optimum nutrition (yet low in calories) our hunger should be satisfied and the diet should not cause nervousness. It should:

Supply Plenty of Energy. If the diet is rich in essential protein amino acids and raw polyunsaturated oils, yet low in carbohydrates, it should supply sustained energy with minimum fluctuations.

Be Rich in Minerals and Trace Minerals. The diet should be rich in natural minerals and trace minerals, and should have a balanced, calcium-phosphorus-magnesium ratio.

Have No Harmful Ingredients. No preservatives—no synthetics—no spray residues—no refined sugar or inorganic bleached flour—no hard fats.

Burn Body Fat. The diet should be designed to burn body fat as well as the oils in the diet.

Be Non-Habit Forming. The diet should not include drugs or habit forming ingredients of any kind.

Be Non-Constipating. The diet should include foods which tend for a soft stool in a natural way. No chemical stool softeners.

Shrink the Intestinal Tract. Contrary to popular opinion that a diet should include plenty of bulk, the diet should be such that there will be a shrinkage of the intestinal tract, in order that the desire for large amounts of food will be lessened, and body dimensions decreased.

Help Digestion. The diet should include raw foods, and additional enzymes to aid proper digestion. Everything should be thoroughly masticated."

For those who wish a quick loss of weight and who

have their doctor's permission, there is a new protein powder which taken four times daily in liquid satisfies all of these requirements.

So forget your crash diets. Choose whichever of these diets which appeals to you most. Begin on this new way of life. You will never be hungry and you should look and feel better than ever before.

20 How to Exercise for Beauty

You can eat the best diet in the world and still not be healthy. And, you have learned by now, if you aren't healthy, you can't be really beautiful.

I have talked with people who were healthy and radiant. "Is nutrition responsible for your good health and good looks?" I asked them.

I knew that these people were devotees of nutrition and I was hoping they would say, "Yes." To my surprise, they said, "No, not entirely." They explained that though responsible for their health and appearance, they had found at least two other needs which must be satisfied for perfect results: exercise and freedom from tension. Of course they were right.

You can eat the right food, take the right vitamins and minerals, but if your circulation is sluggish, your blood stream cannot distribute these goodies to the various parts of your body to sustain or repair them. You can even apply nutritional substances to your face and hair, but without proper circulation they will not be as well assimilated.

You can ruin good health and good looks by tension, but we will discuss how to handle that problem in the next chapter. Let's improve our circulation first.

As you age, your circulation slows down. In youth it is 100 per cent efficient. In old age it may dwindle to 25 per cent. In the ages between there is a gradual decline. Fortunately, there is an easy solution for this problem: exercise.

IS EXERCISE REALLY NECESSARY?

Most people hate to exercise. I am one of them. Yet the rewards are too great to ignore.

Vogue tells of the beauty values of exercise: "A body that gives the impression of vitality, of sleeked-up shape; a body that looks young. As new levels of body tone are established, there is evidence not only of sleekness of leg or firmness of arm, but evidence of *radiant fitness* . . . which lights up the skin, increases strength and goes on to generate new energy.

"Fitness shows in the face. It shows in the way you walk down the street, the way you rise to meet an emergency, in the pulse and in staying power. And of course fitness shows in allure, in the skin, in happiness. . . .

"Efficient exercise can increase almost everyone's capacity. Your performance will increase with use. . . . Exercise produces a feedback of energy, which, working for you on a steady basis, gives you fitness to increase your capacity for vital health and good looks."

An international beauty quoted by *Vogue* adds, "One has always to feel as well as one possibly can, to keep top standards of excellence in health. It takes sleep. It takes discipline. It takes exercise to keep muscle tone. Have you ever seen a woman over forty who looked seductive and who didn't have firm muscles, good health?"

Hans Selye, M.D., the stress expert, mentions a new value of exercise: It helps you to resist stress, something which everyone has these days. To prove this, Dr. Selye took ten unexercised rats and subjected them to all sorts of stress: electric shocks, blinding lights, pain, and loud noises. Within a month they were all dead. Then he took ten other rats and trained them with exercise until they were the equivalent of human long-distance runners. He applied the same stresses to the exercised rats. After a month they were still alive and well.

On the basis of this study Dr. Selye believes that exercise definitely helps nerves resist stress.

Joseph C. Risser, M.D., a specialist in body mechanics, sums up the good effects of exercise: Besides removing fatigue, distributing nutrients to all parts of the body, strengthening muscles, it stimulates the liver, our great chemical laboratory; it encourages deeper breathing and helps rid the body of impurities; and it improves posture as well as bringing a glow of health to the face, skin and eyes, helping you to appear much younger and feel more vital.

WHAT KIND OF EXERCISE IS BEST?

For some reason, men are easier to convert to exercise than women are. Every man secretly wishes he looked like Mr. America, and would exercise with the least encouragement. Women, on the other hand, though they would be happy to look like Miss America, would rather pass by the honor than exercise. It may be that housewives feel they don't *need* exercise—that they work too hard as it is. Everybody needs exercise, including housewives! The reason: exercise and activity are not the same. Just because you are moving around does not mean you are exercising. You may be working under tension, by repeating the same household chores hour after hour, day after day, and using the same muscles over and over again. This creates waste products, whereas exercise brings fresh blood to the body. Together with good nutrition, exercise helps the body to replace and renew worn-out cells.

A woman who makes her living by doing housework helps me a few hours once a week with my house. She tells me she is usually exhausted at the end of each day. I suggested that she do ten minutes of setting-up exercise every morning.

She looked at me as if I had taken leave of my senses. She said tartly, "But I do nothing else *but* exercise!"

I explained that she was using the same muscles over and over, which was tiring, whereas what she needed was stimulating movement. She grudgingly promised to try ten minutes of all-over exercise every morning for one week. At the end of that time she said, "I feel like a different person. My energy holds out longer, now." And she looked much better.

Exercise cannot be a now-and-then thing, either. It must be regular. You may have to fight yourself, but do set up a daily routine and don't allow it to be interrupted. Once you have broken the habit, you're lost.

If you don't have the determination to follow through

on exercise by yourself—and many people haven't—join
a class.

WHAT KIND OF EXERCISE? AND HOW MUCH?

Isometric exercises strengthen muscles, but they do not
stir up your circulation to the point that it sets the blood
running throughout your entire body. Isometrics will not
reach or strengthen the heart or lungs. For this you need
active, moving exercise. Walking, gardening, swimming,
golfing (without a cart), bowling, tennis—whatever *you*
enjoy, to give you that alive, healthy beauty. It is your
vitality that causes heads to turn when you walk into a
room. The healthy, outdoors look wins every time.

There is no substitute for body-moving exercise, particularly in the fresh air, to encourage deep breathing.
R. W. Holderby, M.D., says, "We should get twenty
minutes of exercising daily to the point of perspiration in
order to burn the sludge out of our blood." Walking can
accomplish this.

Many men and women are obtaining enviable figures
by weight-lifting, either at home or in exercise salons.

Alfred Steinberg has written in *Parade* magazine about
Bob Hoffman. Bob has coached and built up many athletes, including those of the Olympic weight-lifting teams.
He believes weight-lifting is for everybody, not just athletes. He says, "You are your own sculptor. You can mold
and shape your body by weight-lifting." He insists everyone, men and women, can be trim and resoundingly
healthy.

Mr. Steinberg, after watching his own son develop
strength, vitality, and a strong trim body by this method,
decided to sneak into the basement when no one was
looking and try out his son's barbells for himself. He was
getting tired of the roll around his middle, his flabby arms
and disappearing chin. He decided that if his son could
develop firm muscles, it was worth a try for him.

He tells what happened.

"The suggested routine required only about ten minutes
every other day, doing ten repetitions of each exercise
with light weights. Surprisingly, there was no tiredness
after each session, but a new, alert, physical self-awareness.
After a few months, suit jackets were growing snug across
the shoulders, two inches had disappeared from my waist,
the double chin had begun firming up.

"Noting these clear improvements, my wife and daughter began to show a lively interest. They had always assumed that weight-lifting was not for women and were surprised to learn that a number of women do exercise in this way."

George R. Bruce, a corrective exercise expert of California, specializes in weight-lifting exercises for women. He is the author of a book *Curves by Bruce*. He has also produced one beauty-contest winner after another, and "done over" flabby housewives so that they are the envy of their friends and bring wolf whistles from men. Barbells and weights are his method of producing this magic. This equipment is available from sports shops and mail-order houses, as well as from special suppliers.

Both Bob Hoffman and George Bruce recognize that true fitness must also involve good nutrition. Bob is a firm believer in lots of protein. He also believes it is never too late to begin exercise.

Bob advises beginners to start by using their barbells slowly. "Train, don't strain," he says. "It took you years to get into your present condition and you will need some time to work out of it. As your outer muscles strengthen, the internal muscles that hold your organs in place and keep them operating efficiently will also improve. At most, three months of training should begin to reward you with improved health and a prouder body."

There is another, easier way to exercise. Rheo H. Blair, a teacher of physical fitness and nutrition for twenty-two years, has trained students who have won nearly one hundred awards in national and worldwide competition. In an article, "Kick Your Way to Health" (*Let's Live* magazine, July, 1967), he writes, "If I had to choose one exercise that would give the greatest benefit in helping maintain the health of the body, it would be the High Kick Exercise.

"The reason is this: Everyone agrees that the most important area of the body is the midsection, which encases the vital organs: the stomach, the intestines, the entire digestive tract, the liver, the pancreas, the kidneys. It is most important that these organs function normally. To function adequately, they must be held in their perfect natural position. . . .

"When the muscles of the abdomen lose their firmness, they stretch, allowing all the important organs to sag. . . . Not only do senior citizens have pot bellies, some children have them, too. We believe that the stomach should be flat!"

He continues, "The back of the thigh is usually so tight that people are unable to bend over and pick up something from the floor. The High Kick Exercise helps all of these conditions. Don't let the simplicity of this exercise allow you to overlook its great benefits. This is how to do it:

"Take off your shoes. Rise on your toes, keep each leg straight, locked at the knee, then kick your right leg as high as you can. Bring it down and kick your left leg as high as possible. Alternate legs until you feel moderately tired. At first, five kicks with each leg is probably enough. Repeat this set of ten total kicks several times during the day. As you become more conditioned and flexible, you will be able to increase the repetitions. Just take it easy at first. Remember some of those muscles haven't been used for years. When you are able to do 50 kicks with each leg (100 total kicks) you will be in much better condition than you are now. You will notice that the exercise stimulates breathing, lung power, endurance. Your muscles will be more supple, your stomach flatter.

"You will find that this High Kick Exercise is enjoyable, most delightful. I have a complete gymnasium built in my home, but I never miss doing this High Kick Exercise. I feel it is a must."

TOO MUCH EXERCISE HARMFUL

Blair also feels that in some cases the body needs some corrective type of exercise, though he feels that a lot of exercise is not necessary and that excess exercise can be very harmful. Instead, he feels that exercise needs to be adjusted to the individual. In many cases he suggests only two or three minutes of exercise a day. This is certainly a revolutionary philosophy—but the successes, he says, speak for themselves.

For the average citizen who does not wish to be a "muscle man," Blair believes that the High Kick Exercise, done 25 times for each leg daily, does more good than two hours of jogging. In his opinion a little exercise is necessary to stir up circulation, whereas too much exercise depletes the body of energy reserve.

Dr. Leo N. Liss, associate professor of podiatry at the University of California San Francisco Medical Center, agrees. He notes that jogging has become more popular than ever since an article, "Aerobics," appeared in the *Reader's Digest*.

"Aerobics simply means building up the body by means of exercise which develops the use of oxygen," he says. "However, the question arises whether jogging or other aerobic exercises might be too severe for the average person.

"There are some people who are physically able to jog or to perform any of the other violent exercises suggested in the article, and others are not. One must be careful not to overtax the body apparatus which supplies oxygen-carrying blood to its many parts.

"For example," says Dr. Liss, "there are some people who have blood vessels which are clogged up with fatty substances—similar to old water pipes which get rusted on the inside. When this happens the blood vessels may be unable to supply muscles with enough blood necessary to perform strenuous exercise.

"Jogging, whether done in position or on a track, requires a great deal of exertion and a large supply of blood to keep muscles active.

"If the muscles are overtaxed, the lack of blood may not only affect extremities such as foot muscles, but also the heart itself.

"However," concludes Dr. Liss, "if you are physically able, jogging will help develop new muscles, provide more strength and may result in making you feel and look in the pink of health."

SPOT EXERCISES

You may add spot exercise to these all-over body exercises. I do not have room to list them here. Whole books are written on the subject. Magazines include them. Newspapers report them. You will find dozens of books to help you at health stores and libraries.

Some women are enthusiastically using a bust developer with excellent results. It is a pink plastic hand exerciser, looking like a large clam shell, held together with a strong spring hinge. Minutes a day does the good work.

But do try the all-over exercise I have mentioned, first. You may find that you won't need spot exercises at all.

HOW IS YOUR POSTURE?

Good posture commands attention. You look your best by standing or sitting proudly. You look dumpy, awkward, and older, if you don't.

Young people start life standing tall. As you age, gravity begins pulling you toward the earth. Old people are often bent over and stooped, merely because they are not strong enough to resist the force of gravity. Nutrition helps. Research shows that calcium strengthens bony structure and helps you to stand up or sit straight, but posture exercises strengthen your muscles.

Royalty is trained to appear regal from infancy. This is not a special right reserved for kings and queens, princes and princesses. You can look regal, too.

Poor posture can cause aches and pains. If you slump, your internal organs can't operate efficiently. Your spine jackknifes, shutting off circulation to vital nerves and other areas. So good posture can improve health as well as appearance. Here are three excellent posture exercises. They will make you proud of your carriage.

Exercise One: This exercise was invented by a woman, who, when she was young, had miserable posture. She had been a sickly child, had an inferiority complex, and admits that she was not very attractive. In her first teenage year her teacher called her attention to her slouching and suggested that she try to overcome it. A physical examination revealed that she had a spinal curvature, so she decided to try to do something about it. She invented the exercise which she practiced faithfully while she sat, stood, or walked. It is not only easy—as you will see in a minute—but it feels good when you try it.

Years later a physician, writing a book on hip and spine diseases, chose this girl for her perfect posture and noted that her spinal curvature had been apparently corrected. This same girl, partly because of her beautiful posture, then became a model for Miss Liberty on the United States Liberty quarter, issued about the beginning of World War I. If you come across one of these rare quarters today, you can see this good posture for yourself. And here is the exercise which produced it:

Put your hands behind your back, arms straight, hands back to back and fingers interlaced. Twist your thumbs first toward your spine, then away from it. You will find it straightens your spine, raises your chest, and pulls in your stomach. Try this while you walk, sit, or stand. It really feels good. The inventor's name: Doris Doscher Baum.

Exercise Two: This exercise comes from Captain W. P. Knowles, of the Institute of Breathing, in London. Captain

Knowles believes that the way you use your lungs controls your health, resistance to disease, even your life span. His world-renowned method of teaching correct breathing has helped over 100,000 people.

His system appears in six little booklets.* In the first, he gives Step One: good posture. He says, "Choose a hard chair. Sit down in it bolt upright. Tuck your elbows into your sides, palms up. With your elbows hugging your sides, draw your arms back as far as they will go. This will bring your shoulder blades together. Lower your hands to your thighs. Let your head and neck relax slightly.

"When you stand, still keep your shoulder blades together, pressing them gently back and down. Let your arms hang loosely at your sides.

"In this position you cannot drop your chest nor distend your abdomen. You will also give free play to the breathing muscles of your chest and diaphragm."

Exercise Three: This comes from Reba and Bonnie Churchill. Find or draw a straight line on the floor. Slip a yardstick *behind* your shoulders, holding onto each end with each hand. Practice walking tall, as you hold this yardstick behind your shoulders and walk a straight line, even if your thighs slightly brush each other.

THAT WONDERFUL SLANT BOARD

"Twenty minutes on a slant board is equivalent to two hours of sleep. If you do this daily, you'll never need a face lift," says Arlene Dahl.

By lying on a slant board with your feet elevated higher than your head, you divert circulation to your head, neck, and face. It takes strain off your muscles and heart. It helps prolapsed organs fall back into their correct positions.

You'll find that it is extremely relaxing and probably the most pleasant experience of your day. It actually will do more for you than that before-dinner cocktail.

You can buy a slant board, or prop up your old ironing board on a box so that your feet are 15 inches higher than your head.

Dr. N. W. Walker, writing in *Let's Live* magazine (August, 1967), says, "One elderly man continued to use his

---

* Capt. W. P. Knowles, M.C.: *Keep Fit by Better Breathing.* Ingleby, Cherry Rise, Chalfont St. Giles, Bucks, England. Send International Postage Coupon for free brochure.

slant board as a regular daily routine and soon discovered many benefits. Among these was a feeling of restful peace which enabled him to get up from the board much refreshed.

"In course of time, he experienced a sense of rejuvenation, and although way up in years, he walks, looks and acts like a man well rejuvenated. His slant board is undoubtedly one of the means which has helped him to appear younger."

Should you have sensations of discomfort, occasionally noticeable in some people long starved for fresh circulation in the upper part of their bodies, begin your slant board program gently. Start with one minute the first day, two minutes the second, gradually increasing the time as desired.

Be sure to keep your slant board set-up, ready to go. If you have to get it out each time you use it, you will avoid using it. Keep it handy so you can drop down on it often for even a few minutes' relaxation. You will feel—and look—invigorated.

21 More Beauty Tips

Every part of your body needs exercise—including your face, your skin, your hair, your eyes. As you get fresh, rich blood to each of these areas, you help rebuild, regenerate, and beautify them more quickly. Here are some techniques which have truly worked wonders.

SKIN EXERCISE PROMOTES BEAUTY

I asked Dr. George A. Wilson, who is long past his seventies, why he had no wrinkles. He said, "Because I exercise my skin."

When I asked him how, he said he got the stiffest brush

he could find and brushed his skin until the fresh blood flooded into it.

Of course I rushed home to try it. I practically scrubbed the skin off my face. I learned by this experience that it is better to start out with a less harsh brush and do it gently at first until your skin has developed resistance. Meanwhile I learned that others were doing skin brushing in different ways. *Vogue* tells about one woman: "She shines. All over. She buffs her skin with loofah, lava, pumice."

The *Good Housekeeping* Beauty Clinic gives another version: "A complexion brush, moistened and stroked over soap, coaxes pores into action, quickens circulation, helps skin renew itself naturally. Using a feathery rotary motion, start at the base of the throat and work from chin to ear level; then down on nose and around nostril wings, finishing on forehead. Rinse dry skin with warm water, then cool; oily skin with hot water, then cold. Rinse thoroughly right up to the hairline. Pat, don't rub, your face dry."

Betty Morales, a co-owner of Organicville Health Center in Los Angeles, tells me that her smooth skin is due to two techniques. Since Betty is the dietitian who supervised the diet of Murray Rose, three-time winner in the Olympics, she is nutrition-minded with a capital N. She not only sells health foods and vitamins and minerals; she takes them herself. And she feeds them liberally to John T. Clark, her business associate.

Betty said, "Besides loading myself with good nutrition on the inside of my body, I skin-brush the outside. I use loofah mitts (a coarse sponge) and stroke my face until it glows, then I add a protein cream." Actually this protein cream is a clear jelly which comes from Mexico. Betty has used it for ten years and says it helps smooth lines away; even absorbs scars. It also tests the correct acidity on the pH scale with Nitrazine paper.

John Clark, Betty's partner, tells about another form of skin exercise. He says, "This secret was learned from the Indians. At bath time, wet your body. Pour a tablespoon of coarse-grind corn meal into your palm and then rub your wet body until the corn meal is used up. Start with your face and cover all areas until you finish with the soles of your feet. The tub or shower will be covered with corn meal, but don't worry; it won't plug the drain. Neither will it wear out your skin. Rinse, dry, and note the silky feeling of your skin."

Another friend, Dorie D'Angelo, a physiotherapist, is

also noted for her beautiful, radiant, wrinkle-free skin, making her look years younger than she is. She is swamped with requests for her secret, which she learned from Pamela Brenton, that amazing, young-looking seventy-year-old woman. Here it is: Morning and night she rubs virgin olive oil on her face. Then she cuts a lemon and pours a few drops of lemon juice into her palm, applying the lemon juice on top of the olive oil until it becomes "tacky." Next she takes salt (sea salt preferably) and rubs it briskly all over her face, even under her eyes. Finally she rinses everything off with cool water, leaving a film of olive oil on her skin.

Vigorous skin-rubbing accomplishes two things: It removes the dead layers of the "scarfskin," or surface skin, and acts as a tonic by stimulating the nerve endings in the skin, increasing skin activity.

EXERCISE FOR YOUR CROWNING GLORY

Hair and scalp can also be exercised. The *Good Housekeeping* Beauty Department says, "Lacklustre hair radiates new shine with a stepped-up program of fresh air, rest and proper diet. A good hair habit for quick results: 100 brush strokes daily. . . . When you're under par, even glowing hair shows it . . . better yet, polish with two brushes."

Massaging vigorously with your fingertips until the scalp glows, then pulling your hair by the fistfuls, helps to exercise hair and scalp, too.

I asked Mr. Francis, the hair expert, if brushing pulls out hair. He answered, "Not usually, unless the hair roots are small from undernourishment, and the weight of pulling is too much. The hair accumulating in your brush is the old hair that is pushed out and replaced by new growth. This is normal shedding. Brushing is one of the 'million-dollar' secrets to healthy, beautiful hair, and it doesn't cost you a cent to do it. Brushing squeezes the tiny oil gland near each root, and allows the brush to carry the oil to the ends.

"Do be careful of the type of brush you use," he warned. "Be sure it is made of natural, not nylon, bristles."

Dr. Agnes Savill, a dermatologist from Glasgow, Scotland, reported in the *British Journal of Dermatology* that nylon brushes—particularly those with harsh, square-cut bristles—tore out hair by the roots. Under a microscope, Dr. Savill says, the hair was split and looked like a twig.

Brushes made of natural bristles, on the other hand, are kind to the hair. Dr. Savill reports that when natural brushes were used in denuded spots, new hair grew in again.

John W. King, B.Sc., says, "A hair normally has a life of between two and six years. The old hairs are more apt to fall in the spring and early summer, because a person's bodily resistance is usually lower at those seasons. Since hairs do not last a lifetime, it is only natural that a few should fall every day, and if they fall a little oftener in the spring it is nothing to be perturbed about, for they will be replaced with new hairs, provided your scalp is healthy and the resistance of your body normal.

"Regular brushing is one of the finest methods of improving the health of the scalp. A healthy lustre is imparted to the hair, and the papillae, nerves and oil glands of the roots are kept in good condition. The hair shaft and scalp are cleansed of dust and scales. But the most important thing that brushing does is to strengthen the small muscles at the base of each hair. If these muscles are strengthened by brushing, they are able to hold the individual hairs longer."

One New York City salon which prides itself on producing beautiful tresses is owned by a Leningrad-born, medically educated hair specialist, George Michael. Twelve thousand women come to him regularly. Eight thousand have hair below the shoulders. Four thousand have hair below the waist. Eighteen have hair to their knees, and two have hair 7½ feet long.

George Michael says, "Most hair grows six inches per year. The average length of my clients' hair is forty-four inches." He encourages long hair. Why? The longer the hair, the stronger the root, he says.

How does he produce so many heads of magnificent tresses? He recommends a shampoo such as a neutral castile-like soap; 200 strokes of brushing (no cheating), brushing upward from the hair-line, and *diet!*

This man knows what he is talking about. He wrote his first thesis on hair in 1941. His clients are proof that his system works.

THE MAN WHO THREW AWAY HIS GLASSES

One friend, a professional man, tells me that he has recovered his health as a result of nutrition. One night after a convention in a Chicago hotel, I sat between him and another man who has achieved good health through corrected nutrition. I swiveled my head from one to the other, much like watching a tennis match, as each man told of the ailments which had departed once and for all as a result of using nutritional therapy. The combined list included an ulcer, hemorrhoids, constipation, sinus trouble, indigestion, high cholesterol, a serious form of heart disturbance, arthritis, and other assorted problems. Each man seemed to top the other with an account of his ailments. Both men are now pictures of perfect health.

The first man won the tournament, at least for the evening, by telling how he achieved good eyesight and threw away his glasses. Here is his story:

"In 1948 it became necessary for me to get glasses. I was twenty at the time. My health was considered 'average' although I had chronic sinus and ear trouble. At the time I was also working under fluorescent lighting in a bank, which meant I was involved in writing and working with figures. I began suffering a 'pulling' sensation in and around my eyes and also had very frequent headaches, which would gradually disappear after working hours.

"I consulted my physician, who referred me to an eye specialist. It was determined by examination that I was near-sighted in one eye, farsighted in the other eye, had simple astigmatism and muscle weakness that prevented proper focusing. Glasses were prescribed.

"In the following seven years my lenses were changed to stronger ones twice, making three separate prescriptions in all. I had changed my work, but still worked under fluorescent fixtures although no figures or writing were involved.

"It was in the seventh year that my symptoms appeared again. I immediately consulted my eye doctor. He could find no need to change the prescription and appeared puzzled. He tightened my frames and checked the prescription carefully and suggested that the difficulty was physical. My physician denied this.

"Why the change? Why the recurrence of symptoms? I began thinking about this problem. I could find nothing significant. I then considered trying nutrition. My next step was to get books on nutrition and check them for items about eyes and eye care.

"*Let's Eat Right to Keep Fit*, by Adelle Davis, was full

of help. It mentions twenty-one eye dysfunctions and problems related to nutrition! Next I checked my intake of vitamins and minerals. One answer was obviously there. With hope and optimism I again contacted my eye doctor, who told me diet had nothing to do with my problem, and I believed him. I did not know at the time that his training did not include a course in nutrition.

"Nevertheless, I began taking special supplements daily. In less than one month the change was so dramatic that the eye doctor said, "Well, there just might be something to it," and began giving me exercises with the aid of a machine in his office. In another month I threw the glasses away. This was in 1955 and my eyes are excellent today! (1968) This is what I did to accomplish this 'miracle'!

"I firmly believe that relaxation and circulation are basic keys to eye health if proper nutrients are available to nourish the eye. As for fluorescent lighting, I read *My Ivory Cellar*, by Dr. John Ott, which reports disturbing results from such lighting. I am glad I started avoiding it years ago.

"Next, eye exercises: The exercises in the eye specialist's office gave me an idea. I exercised at home one minute per day, regularly, in the morning when I was less fatigued. I sat in a chair placed against the center of a wall of a square room. I placed my head against the wall to assure no head movement. I looked at the high corner of the room where the wall meets the ceiling. I then moved my eyes slowly from one corner to the other (left to right, and right to left). This slow, deliberate movement does exercise the eye and a few trials will prove this to you. It is simple, but effective.

"Third, relaxation. We all know what it is, but how many attain relaxation? Coffee, tea, smoking, and stimulants constrict the blood vessels. We hurry all day. We are exposed to obvious and subtle tension factors (radio, street noise, television, etc.). We must make a conscious effort to relax. Body exercise, too, like relaxation, aids all health!

"Fourth, nutrition. If we can relax and stimulate circulation through exercise, then the nutrients in the blood naturally aid the body in maintaining health or rebuilding it. This is a basic fact. For eyes, it appears that the prime nutrients for problems are B-complex vitamins, vitamin C (with rutin and bioflavonoids) and vitamin A. (Remember that I am not prescribing, but only relating my experience.) I used 25,000 IU (International Units) of vitamin A each morning before breakfast with 10 grains of calcium lactate. After breakfast I took a vitamin B complex tablet and the vitamin C tablet (which contains 350 mg. of ascorbic acid, 50 mg. of rutin, 350 mg. of bioflavonoids, plus 10 mg. of hesperidin complex).

"After lunch I took another vitamin B and vitamin C tablet.

"Nutrition plus the eye exercise returned my eyes to normal."

HELP FOR A PRETTIER NECK

Here are some exercises for a firm chin line.

Vogue says, "Play at being Eve. Dangle the reddest, roundest, most succulent apple in the world over your head (in your imagination).

"Tip your head back; hold your arms down, relax your shoulders and reach for that apple. Use only the muscles of your throat and neck and pull, pull, pull toward that apple.

"The apple may be imaginary, the results aren't; stronger looking throat; neck visibly longer and supple; good firm tone to the band of muscles under your chin."

Fifi D'Orsay, a former movie star, says, "All the women in my family get what we call 'robin's throat,' a kind of double chin. I decided very young that *I* was going to keep my contour! I never missed exercising every night and wouldn't go to sleep until I did my routine. My muscles are still firm. Here is the exercise:

"Drop your head forward, chin resting on your chest (you are in a sitting position). Leading with your chin, come up to a position so that you are looking at the ceiling. Drop your jaw, let your chin protrude until you feel a strong pull in the neck muscles. Slowly but forcefully, bring your lower teeth over your upper lip and upper teeth. Do this about ten times nightly. When done correctly the under-chin area is given a firm work-out."

DO-IT-YOURSELF FACE LIFT

Many women have been disappointed in their use of cosmetics because they somehow expected a face lift that did not materialize. We've learned that certain cosmetics applied to the skin can certainly improve its surface, but sagging contours, flabbiness, jowls, and drooping eyelids are not due to surface causes. Muscles that are weakened can no longer hold their original position in the facial contours, and when they sag, it adds years to the appearance.

To make things worse, other facial imperfections develop and show up as the muscles let down. Wrinkles, crow's-feet, under-eye bags, distended neck cords, and other faults become apparent and worsen with each passing year.

Until a short time ago, there seemed to be only two alternatives for maturing women and men. One was to accept the fact and fate of a dismally unattractive future of looking increasingly older and uglier, or resort to plastic surgery, which is both temporary and expensive. Now, thanks to a new and scientifically exacting program, neither is necessary.

Every so often in history someone comes along and solves a problem that has bothered people for ages. For example, dry skin treatment: women have used creams on their faces almost since the beginning of time, hoping to ward off drying and aging. Then, in this twentieth century it was discovered that not cream alone, but moisture incorporated with cream, gave better results. So moisturizers were developed and are now a household cosmetic used by discerning men and women the world over.

Also, just recently in this century, the problems of delaying and changing sagging facial contours has been solved. It is an established fact that flabby body muscles can be reconditioned and made firm and supple again through exercise. Since the flesh of the face and neck is supported by muscles, it, too, can be made to return almost to its original firmness and youthful contours by properly done exercises that restore muscle tone. People have waited for this kind of good news for ages.

The concept of facial-muscle exercising is not entirely new. Several people have experimented with it earlier, but the method was often vague, both to the investigators and to the women who tried it. Isometric exercises, which enjoyed a flurry of popularity, were also tried. These, too, produced less than satisfactory results. Several researchers who made a thorough study of facial anatomy and spent many years in research have developed a scientifically exacting method of exercising the face and neck. It really works!

Various people are responsible for this wonderfully encouraging outlook, and they have proved that women and men no longer need dread looking old. The program that they have developed not only prevents facial aging, but it helps to reverse wrinkles, scowl lines, sagging, and other discouraging faults.

One researcher says, "Nature's way of renewing the body is through blood circulation. Exercise brings a fresh blood supply to the area, stimulating and giving tone to the skin and muscles and creating a healthier condition from the inside out! Exacting and specifically developed exercises help the muscles gain more tone and firmness. These muscles then pull up sagging cheeks and chins; to eliminate puffiness under eyes; and to mellow frown creases and laugh lines. Exercises alone won't work the miracle of rejuvenation; they must be scientifically coordinated with resistance."

Because there has been such a great demand for simple but effective face exercises, I have compiled a small book which contains the findings of some experts on face anatomy and face re-education. This book, called *Face Improvement Through Exercise and Nutrition** is easy to understand and use. It is true that unless you practice improvement exercises of any kind consistently, you cannot expect results. But this book is made so easy for you that a few minutes a day, used as automatically as you brush your teeth, can definitely improve your appearance. Either in the morning before you apply your makeup, or at night when you take it off, a few minutes of bringing fresh circulation through exercise to the areas which are slipping can really help. These facial exercises, used regularly and effortlessly, and adapted to your own way of life, can also prevent signs of aging before they start. Even after these signs of aging have arrived, they can be reversed, as confirmed by two experts who tried them on themselves after the age of seventy, with surprising results. (The results are described in my book.)

Many movie and TV stars, men and women alike, practice this type of exercise daily. One woman who used them was asked by her friends, "What have you been doing? Have you been on a vacation? You have never looked so well."

Face-lifts help temporarily but often must be repeated. You can help your own face to lift and stay lifted by a small

---

*New Canaan, Conn. Keats Publishing Inc. Paperback. 1973.

investment of time spent daily on a few simple exercises designed to improve the whole face or problem areas only. It is a rewarding habit to include in your self-improvement program.

Many doctors do not believe face-lifting (cosmetic surgery) is always necessary. If they do recommend it, they believe that strengthening the face through exercise brings better results or help in later muscle control.

Beauty experts recommend facial exercises as do dentists who encourage facial rehabilitation in denture or orthodontia patients.

My book, *Face Improvement Through Exercise and Nutrition*, shows how to accomplish good results by combining exercises and good nutrition. The book includes "how-to" illustrations for the reader to follow. Every person should exercise the face as regularly as one brushes hair or teeth, or jogs or does push-ups. It pays off when a friend or family member says, "You look great!"

Meanwhile, there is a form of instant face lift you can use the rest of your life: A smile!

22 How to Handle Tensions

Tension can interfere with health. Hans Selye, M.D., the stress expert, explains why: In prolonged stress, you unconsciously tense an area of your body—gall bladder, kidneys, even your heart area—without realizing it. Tension will thus prevent proper circulation and normal delivery of nutrients to, or assimilation by, that organ, eventually leading to organ starvation, stagnation, malfunction, and disease.

As a result of tension, digestion also slows down or

ceases, inhibiting the manufacture of hydrochloric acid and other digestive fluids. Food is not assimilated. Adding HCL or other digestants can, of course, help the digestion, but not eliminate mealtime tension. Bickering, quarreling, talking about unpleasant subjects can play havoc with digestion. One woman with whom I lunch now and then orders her lunch, then settles down with grim satisfaction to list all the operations, diseases, and deaths among her friends. To her, this must be relaxing. As for me, I can actually feel my stomach muscles curl up in a knot.

These are tense times. Few people are immune to worry or tension. It is more than ever necessary to do something to avoid its impact, else it will disturb the body. Dr. Selye feels that stress can lead to, or be the cause of, all manner of diseases, including ulcers, arthritis, high blood pressure, constricted blood vessels, and heart ailments. Cancer has even been linked with stress and depression. All this would sound far-fetched if it were not for Dr. Selye's explanation that a tensed body resists absorbing the life-renewing fresh blood and the nutrients it carries for self-repair. We must do something to outwit tensions. Fortunately, it is possible.

Everyone has problems. There is no avoiding them. However, it is not the problem, but how you face it, that counts. Sometimes, though, problems appear insoluble. There is no place to turn, it seems; no help available. At this point most people gulp tranquilizers or sleeping pills, consume cartons of cigarettes or unlimited alchohol. These do not solve the problem: they merely anesthetize the mind of the person who is facing it and make him less able to cope with the situation. There are better ways to handle tension.

NUTRITIONAL HELP FOR MIND AND BODY

Emotional tensions are increasing, while most people's bodies are weakening. Dr. Heinz Lehmann, of McGill University, Montreal, says, "We are more hurried than our parents were; we are also probably exposed to much greater stimulation than we were originally constructed for."

We are also less nutritionally fortified than our ancestors.

A weak body can make the mind ill. Many mental disturbances have cleared up as if by magic when certain nutrients were fed to the body. Freud himself has stated that mental ills in the future will respond to the ministrations of the biochemist—the specialist who sets the body chemistry in order by providing certain nutrients. This prediction is already coming true. Many people who are depressed, nervous, even considered candidates for psychiatric care or mental institutions, have recovered *completely* when a nutritionally observant doctor found that their mental disturbance was due to a physical disturbance, hypoglycaemia (low blood sugar). This bodychemistry disturbance can be reversed, not by drugs, psychiatric measures or confinement, but by *a simple diet*.

Another mental-emotional aberration, schizophrenia, responds to a vitamin, niacin or nicotinic acid, also called vitamin B-3. Cases have been reported in which people who were suspicious, almost psychotic, have recovered within hours after being given this B vitamin. Two psychiatrists have tested it thoroughly and written about its value in emotional disturbances. This book is *How to Live with Schizophrenia*, by Abram Hoffer, M.D., Ph.D. and Humphry Osmond, M.R.C.S., D.P.M.

Although this team of psychiatrists used one vitamin only, nutritionally trained physicians would include *all* nutritional substances for even better results.

Perhaps the reason that nutrition helps to prevent or correct stress conditions in the body or mind is that it helps to provide a built-in resistance against stimuli and worry. A weak body does not resist stress as well as a strong one. Recall the old phrase, "A strong mind in a strong body."

Tranquilizers, pep pills and barbiturates merely mask, not correct, emotional tensions. Safe nutritional substances include calcium, lecithin, the entire vitamin B complex (including niacin), and vitamin C. After a shock of *any* kind—news of a death, a mortgage due, or even an argument with husband or wife—the vitamin C reserve stored in your adrenal glands is exhausted within minutes. By replacing vitamin C in massive doses, the normal level in the body is restored. Vitamin C protects against infection and other disturbances. Researchers have now learned that many colds occur after an emotional problem because the protective vitamin C has been destroyed, leaving a clear pathway to infection. Some forms of cancer have now been shown to follow worry, perhaps for the same reason: one of the body's protective or repair nutrients has been destroyed and not replaced.

THE EFFECT OF MIND ON BODY

A disturbed emotional condition can throw health out of balance and cause almost unbelievable physical repercussions. A friend of mine, a man, began to be troubled with abdominal cramps so severe that he actually rolled on the floor with excruciating pain. His family doctor could find no physical cause. He tried various medications, which provided only temporary relief. The painful cramps continued.

One day the doctor asked his patient when the cramps had begun. Together the two men traced the beginning back two months. "Did anything change in your work or home at that time?" the doctor asked.

Light dawned in the man's eyes. "My mother-in-law came for a prolonged visit. She has been ordering me around ever since," he said.

When the mother-in-law's visit was terminated abruptly by the man's wife, at the request of the doctor, the cramps disappeared and never returned. Professional help is undeniably useful in such unexplained situations.

RELAXATION DISSOLVES TENSION

Frances Lucile Kraft, Ph.D., is an expert in teaching the technique of deliberate relaxation. She says, "Training in relaxation is not a panacea, but it is an important and effective means of improving one's health status. . . . We, as individuals, cannot do very much to reform the world or retard its accelerating pace, but we can [learn how to] offset the tension-producing effects by changing ourselves and conserving our energy."

THE RAG-DOLL EXERCISE

The rag-doll type of relaxation program was tried by volunteers in a hospital. The instructions were broadcast over the public-address system. Those who followed the suggestions reported that the technique helped them rest better and sleep better, and feelings of anxiety were lessened.

Briefly, here is my condensed version of the general method:

1. Slowly bend or stiffen your right foot. Relax. Then

your right calf. Relax. Next, your right thigh. Relax.

2. Repeat with the other leg. As you relax each segment, maintain the relaxation throughout the entire 45-minute session until the entire body is relaxed.

3. Tense your abdomen. Relax.

4. Tense and relax each arm, in sections as you did your legs: hand, upper arm, forearm.

5. Tense and relax the lung area. Breathe deeply several times.

6. Tense and relax your shoulders. Drop them.

7. Tense your neck. Circle your head several times, rotating first to one side, then the other. Drop your chin to your chest. This is one area where most people are tense.

8. Tense your face. Tense your mouth, your jaw, your chin, relaxing each in turn. Squeeze your eyes shut and relax. Raise your eyebrows.

Somewhere in this process you will discover areas of tension you had not previously noticed. Every hour on the hour, even at work, check each part of your body quickly to spot residual tension and relax. This check-up will take but a few seconds.

This relaxation method is also excellent for insomnia. As you lie on your back in bed you will often fall asleep before you complete your "rag-doll exercise."

Curtis Mitchell sums up, "Tension is a habit. Substitute another habit—relaxing. Every time you practice, it helps. At first your mind will wander, fuss, and fume. Follow through. Tension is doing something; relaxing is doing nothing. Relaxation lengthens muscles. In relaxing, your muscles learn to relax, your nervous system relaxes, and nature takes over to heal and invigorate.

"The method is easy. Use it to erect a bulwark against personal illness, tension, inefficiency. The cost is a fragment of time and a jot of your will power. The reward is beyond description."

One of the greatest bonuses of such a relaxation program is a more beautiful face. Arlene Dahl in her beauty column says, "Responsibility for both serene complexions and dispositions are the daily beauty siestas of South-of-the-Border women. They relax for about 20 minutes in solitude after lunch and before dinner."

Sleep is also healing. It calms nerves, helps problems fade into their proper perspective. I have fully covered the subject of insomnia in my book, *Get Well Naturally*. There are documented reports that B vitamins taken daily, honey, a teaspoonful at bedtime; or calcium tablets, are far safer than sleeping pills. They do not leave you groggy or muddle-headed the next day, have no side effects, and are not habit-forming. Most insomniacs I know keep a bottle of calcium tablets—any kind—on their bedside table, together with a glass of water, to use as needed.

Sleep is also beautifying. Dolores Del Rio, the movie star of many years ago, is considered as beautiful today as she was at the height of her career. She attributes her beauty to sleep, sleep, sleep.

YOU ARE WHAT YOU THINK

One woman said, "After ten years of living with a hopeless alcoholic, my face shows everything I've lived through—mouth drooping, heavy nose-to-mouth lines. Gloom, worry, depression have left their mark."

Facial muscles definitely react to thoughts and emotions. Dr. Rose Le Fohn, who produces the famous mink-oil cosmetics, says, "Every line in your face reflects your mental attitude. If you think, 'I am growing old,' you will grow old rapidly. Each day must be approached with gratitude for the new day in your life. Each day must be approached with courage and with enthusiasm. You cannot progress without the enthusiasm factor. Learn to ignore petty annoyances. Cultivate an eagerness for some new hobby or soul-absorbing work that breaks down the barriers of your life. In short, learn to side-step or put yourself out of the way of irritations. The thing you are trying to accomplish will be done as if by a miracle."

Doris Day adds, "Diet, exercise, and cosmetics all are part of looking and feeling well. But if a woman wants to be healthy-looking and vital, the main thing is to think right."

HOW TO SOLVE PROBLEMS

One practicing psychologist who has taught hundreds of students how to be successful says the trick of accomplishing something which you wish to do, or a chore which bothers you, is easy. *Just visualize it as being done!* If it is your house you want to clean, yet dread cleaning it, make a mental picture of it shining and clean. If it is a report you must write, visualize it as finished, and see yourself turning it in. The subconscious accepts a picture, and uses it as a blueprint for accomplishment. Thus it can ease your load, smooth your way, speed your efforts.

The technique can help you become healthier and more beautiful. As you go to sleep at night, make a picture of how you want to look, how you want to feel. See others congratulating you on your appearance. See yourself looking and acting and feeling buoyant, radiant, alive, vital. Give yourself suggestions such as, "I am beginning to feel better, and look better. I *do* look better. I *do* feel better." This, combined with imagery or visualization, is the secret of many a beautiful, healthy, and successful person. It is the effortless way.

Here is another affirmation:

> I am well, strong and vital
> I am beautiful, pure and good
> I am on the road to eternal youth
> Pure red blood is running through my body
> Removing all obstruction
> Bringing peace, health and harmony.
>   Author unknown

SPIRITUAL VITAMINS

There is a higher power directing us, as it created us, *if we ask for help.* One minister friend of mine says, "You need ask only once. After asking, continue to give thanks that the solution is coming. There is a way out of everything, if you ask for help."

Adela Rogers St. John, the author, believes that people who pray for guidance usually do not wait for an answer. They tell God what to do, instead of waiting for God to tell them. She states that when she is faced with a problem, large or small, she immediately asks for divine help. Then she waits for an answer. It may come in different ways: through a person, a phone call, a book, a letter, or by some other route. It may not come instantly. It rarely comes in the manner one expects. Patience is important. But it comes, she states firmly, if you are sincere and willing to wait for the answer.

Often, while she waits, she thumbs through the Bible. Suddenly a flash of understanding or knowledge will come; or the Bible will open almost of itself to a passage which holds the solution.

Meanwhile, count your blessings, not your woes, to help the blessings to multiply.

You need no longer be at the mercy of difficult events. Rise above them, sidestep them, ask for help and give thanks that your petition has been heard and that help is on the way. These are spiritual vitamins.

23 How to Be Beautiful

Some people are born beautiful. Others *make* their beauty. This is nothing new. It began with Cleopatra.

One of the most beautiful women I know attracts admiring glances wherever she goes. Men swoon over her. Women sigh with envy. She has been chosen as a national symbol of a well-known product, advertised from coast to coast. She has been a model. She has appeared on radio, television, and the stage. She also is a wife and mother. Even though I have long counted her as one of my most cherished friends, I had always assumed that she had been born beautiful. One day I learned differently.

I stopped at her house early one morning and caught her before she completed her beauty routine for the day.

Her head was wrapped in a turban. I learned later that it was helping her hair absorb an application of raw, beaten egg prior to a shampoo, and that she tinted it herself with a natural, safe coloring. When I interrupted her she was working in the garden and her turban was topped with a large sun hat. Her arms were covered with long sleeves. To my astonishment, instead of a flawless skin, I found that her face was sprinkled with a liberal supply of freckles, giving her a pixie expression. She explained, "Being a redhead, I cannot allow the sun to touch my face and arms or I become a mass of freckles."

Her usually beautiful, luminous eyes were now un-made-up, and her brows and lashes were pale and uninteresting. She looked like an ordinary mortal. I was dumbfounded.

Later I asked for her beauty secrets, which she generously shared with me.

She is a strong believer in natural substances, used both internally and externally. She believes true beauty is always based on good health. Beautiful hair and good health do not "just happen." Therefore, she keeps her health, the fine texture of her skin and hair, through proper nutrition, inside and out.

Although she started life not actually as an ugly duckling, she was one who might easily have been lost in a crowd. She learned how to acquire beauty by minimizing her liabilities, maximizing her assets. Through modeling, she learned how to wear clothes and carry herself proudly. Her beautiful voice was developed through voice training. Through stage and television experience she learned the art of make-up. It appears so natural it is scarcely noticeable. Many women have started life with far more beauty assets and accomplished fewer results.

This woman has something more than superficial beauty: she has an inner, shining personality which lights up her eyes and warms her smile. She is sweet, loving, outgoing, and genuinely interested in everyone. Consequently, she is loved by all who know her. She is also devoutly religious, which adds the glow of a beautiful spirit to her acquired beauty.

So beauty can be acquired; it can also be lost. I am reminded of a movie star who, as a country teenager, was "discovered" through photographs. Because she was too young to have learned the secrets of camouflage, her beauty was apparently natural, not acquired.

Several years after being groomed by the studios, she became one of the great beauties of the screen. Then, little by little, she became disillusioned with success and four unsuccessful marriages. Public acclaim bored her. Columnists began to report her incessant drinking, smoking, use of drugs. She stayed until the wee hours in night clubs. Gradually her beauty began to fade. Today, though she is exactly the same age of my friend, who is still healthy and looks beautiful, that movie star's natural beauty is gone. Her skin and hair have lost their sheen. With dark circles and bags beneath her eyes, she looks old and haggard. She is resentful over her lost beauty and wears an expression of bitterness. She is avoided by everyone who formerly courted her.

YOU MUST WORK AT BEING BEAUTIFUL

Count Marco, the San Francisco *Chronicle* columnist, tells of overhearing women discussing a beautiful woman. They say, "Oh, she's so beautiful, she doesn't have to do much to herself."

He disagrees. "The more beautiful a woman is, the more others expect from her and the more time she has to spend on herself. You have to work at being a beauty," he concludes.

The beautiful model Suzy Parker agrees. She feels that you can't get your hands or skin or hair in condition in ten minutes or ten days. You have to work at it all the time—it takes a lot of planning, a little daily doing, and a combination of wise food, sound sleep, comfortable feet, and daily exercise and relaxation. If you plan it, you can do it, she says. Then when the phone rings and a friend says, "How soon can you join us?" you are basically ready—all but final dressing and make-up. This way you will never be caught with anything but your good looks showing.

Nancy Reagan, wife of California's governor, Ronald Reagan, was asked by the beauty editor of a woman's magazine how she always managed to look marvelous and completely at ease. Mrs. Reagan admitted that her main secret is to be so well organized that her clothes, skin, and hair are always in good condition. She maintains a daily beauty ritual. She uses as little make-up as possible, but what cosmetics she does use are made of natural substances.

An athlete must remain in rigid training to succeed. His diet and sleep are strictly supervised by his coach, who knows that incorrect eating, insufficient sleep and exercise can add up to a poor performance record. Smoking and alcohol are banned. Those who take part in the Olympic Games are forbidden to use drugs such as pep pills and tranquilizers because they have been found to be hazardous to good performance.

Few athletes suffer from the usual aches and pains experienced by others. They sleep like babies. Their appearance and vitality are magnetic.

To remain successful, movie and television stars must follow a similar plan. They know that improper food, drinking, smoking, and late hours show up in figures and faces before the relentless cameras. Like athletes, they must keep constantly in training or lose out. Yet those who value their health and appearance would not trade this way of life for the self-indulgence of their dissolute colleagues who lose their health, their looks, their audience, and eventually their jobs.

Look at Robert Cummings, Gloria Swanson, Marlene Dietrich as examples of those who adhere to a regular, daily training program.

Actually a program for beautification is not as hard as it sounds. Once set up, it becomes automatic, like brushing your teeth or driving a car; though creating beauty is more exciting, rewarding, and fun.

Everyone has an audience. It may be your family, your friends, your community to which you are constantly on display. You need to build and maintain an image of beauty and never let your audience down. For example, wearing curlers to the supermarket is just as disillusioning to shoppers as it is to your husband.

Preparation is undeniably necessary in order to maintain your beauty image, but all beauty rituals should be conducted behind the scenes. Choose a time for them when your family is away from home, or choose a sanctuary such as the bathroom where you will not be interrupted until you are ready to appear at your best. Choose moisturizers which don't show for night use. Wear an attractive turban to hide your curlers. Wear something attractive (including make-up) first thing in the morning. Make your family as well as your friends proud of your appearance.

There is nothing which contributes more to good morale than to know that *at all times,* whether it is for the benefit of the milkman or the VIP your husband unexpectedly brings home for dinner, *you are looking your best.* A program well-planned and followed every day without exception will make this possible. Actually your plan will soon become so automatic that you will eat the right things, without a second thought. You will suddenly realize with surprise that compliments from others indicate your beauty plan is paying off.

Don't give in to discouragement. There will be good days and bad days, but it is the long run which counts.

Some people are so concerned over their liabilities that they forget their assets. They become obsessed with some fault and, in their minds, it assumes importance out of all proportion. For example, several people have said, "If I only had a different nose, I could be beautiful." After endless agonizing they resorted to plastic surgery and acquired a different-shaped nose, only to report, "Nobody noticed the difference!"

Remember that 99 per cent of all people have one or more physical defects. They also have at least one physical asset, usually more. The solution is to improve, minimize, or camouflage the faults, then detour attention around to the assets. I know a woman whose figure is far from perfect. But her skin and hair are so beautiful (and she *made* them that way) people don't even notice her figure; only her skin and hair.

Many women have gone down in history as beauties. When they were analyzed, their beauty was not due to perfection of face or figure at all. Instead, their reputation was earned for warmth, sympathy, and interest in others. And this proves a point: We should make ourselves as beautiful as we can; but this should not be a narcissus-like goal or a nonstop self-absorption with beauty. Beauty should not be a goal in itself, but a means to an end.

You can have perfect features, a perfect figure, and still not be beautiful. Look in any store window at a mannequin. You will see perfection of skin, figure, posture, hair arrangement, make-up, and even clothes. But as you look at that mannequin's face, it is cold; it lacks the warmth of a smile, or a loving expression in the eyes.

Once you have achieved a beautiful exterior through your health-and-beauty plan, *forget about yourself.* Turn your attention, your interests, your sympathy and love to others, as you would wish them to react to you. As you allow this inner radiance to shine through your eyes and your smile, you will, in turn, become truly beautiful. This is the real secret of beauty: a beauty of spirit, that quality for which the beauties extolled through the ages are remembered forever.

Eleanore King writes:* "Fortunately, the skills for laying a sound basis of habit are teachable, learnable, masterable. Fortunately also, you can apply them as you go about your daily work. You weave them into your life. You learn through doing. You move gracefully until that is your only way of movement. You incorporate radiant, sincere facial expressions until they become yours. You

* From *Guide to Glamor,* Englewood Cliffs, N.J. (Prentice-Hall, 1937).

practice tactful, gracious conversation until any other kind would be foreign to you. Saying cheerful, encouraging words influences your thinking. Words help thoughts, and thoughts help words. They stamp you indelibly.

"Soon your friends, your business associates, even your family notice, first, a subtle change, then a remarkable one. Then you hear, 'You're a glorious person.' And you are. You willed yourself to be. You won't succumb to the pettiness and self-pity which are all too often the props of those who justify their laziness with alibis. You will continue your steady progress forward in the ranks of happy, loving, successful people.

"I have watched the meekest become confident; the dullest, gay; the most awkward, graceful; the plain, radiant; the defeated, victorious; the discouraged, confident; the miserable, happy. Those with only the usual worries, slight in comparison, were cinches to be successes. They couldn't lose.

"Never criticize *anyone*, either to his face or behind his back. You will instantly lose the confidence of your admirers. Bless, or praise, instead. If you cannot say anything pleasant, say nothing at all. A critical attitude makes enemies, not friends, and destroys the illusion of beauty.

"You will become a finer person when you recognize that you wish to live in harmony with God's laws. Laws of love, mercy, patience, forbearance, tolerance, joy. You will live on the side of the virtues of wisdom, understanding, counsel, fortitude, knowledge and piety. They are for you. They will be the basis for your way of life. You know that with these possessions you will be happy, cheerful, friendly, outgiving. Their presence is gentle and unmistakable. Your family and friends will respond in turn. You will begin to generate a warmth, a radiance, that will draw people to you. You will be truly beautiful."

A NEW YOU

When you begin your make-over program, don't become impatient. Your body may need weeks, perhaps months, to regenerate itself. A hit-or-miss program will not work, only a consistent program will bring rewards.

The results will not come overnight or even be sustained at first. You will have a good day now and then in which you feel more energetic. This is a sign that the repair materials are beginning to do their job. Perhaps the next day may seem a failure, possibly because the nutrients have been used up and need to be replaced. Fill up your reservoir and keep it full of these wonderful rebuilding factors. Use them on your skin and hair, too.

Make this plan automatic, a way of life. Before too long you will suddenly realize that the benefits are increasing.

This rebuilding program, which includes correct nutrition used inside and out, plus exercise, relaxation, and right thinking, is the direct route to health and beauty. Others have found it successful. So can you.

Best of Luck!

Index